Practice Supervision and Assessment in Nursing, Health and Social Care

T0256286

This is an essential guide for all health and social work practitioners supporting an increasing number of learners, trainees, apprentices and pre-registration students engaging in practice-based and work-based learning. Applying educational learning theory to underpin the role and practice of the contemporary practice supervisor, assessor and educator, this accessible book presents strategies for practice learning and personal development.

Acknowledging the problematic nature of learning within the workplace, the authors place the lived experience of the learner at the heart of this text and emphasise the critical importance of an expansive and compassionate learning environment for all. The book includes chapters on the context of practice learning, the role of the supervisor/assessor and educator, learning environments, coaching, assessment and supporting the learner in difficulty, among others. It also spotlights practice learning in a range of settings, from working with children, through social care and maternity care. Each chapter includes learning outcomes and activities, as well as a chapter summary.

Designed for nurses, midwives, social workers, therapists and operating department practitioners who support learners in the workplace, this text is particularly relevant to registrants completing practice supervisor/assessor/educator preparation and pre-registration students taking modules on supporting learning.

Dr Mark Wareing (editor) completed his nurse training at the Birmingham College of Nurse Education and held a number of posts in medicine and surgery before establishing the specialist urological nursing service in North Oxfordshire as a clinical nurse specialist employed by the Department of Urology in Oxford. Prior to entering education, Mark served for four years as a captain in the Reserve Army Medical Services and was deployed to Iraq in 2004. He was a lecturer and senior lecturer in health and social care at Birmingham City University until 2015. As a principal lecturer and director of practice learning at the University of Bedfordshire, Mark provided academic leadership relating to practice learning across HCPC and NMC approved and commissioned healthcare courses across the Faculty of Health and Social Sciences. He was appointed reader and department director of practice education at Brunel University London in July 2023.

Practice Supervision and Assessment in Nursing, Health and Social Care

Edited by Mark Wareing

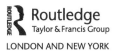
Routledge
Taylor & Francis Group

LONDON AND NEW YORK

Cover design credit: © Getty Images

First published 2025
by Routledge
4 Park Square, Milton Park, Abingdon, Oxon OX14 4RN

and by Routledge
605 Third Avenue, New York, NY 10158

Routledge is an imprint of the Taylor & Francis Group, an informa business

British Library Cataloguing-in-Publication Data
A catalogue record for this book is available from the British Library

ISBN: 978-1-032-41541-3 (hbk)
ISBN: 978-1-032-41538-3 (pbk)
ISBN: 978-1-003-35860-2 (ebk)

DOI: 10.4324/9781003358602

Typeset in Optima
by MPS Limited, Dehradun

Contents

Figures

Tables

Introduction

Mark Wareing

Registered health and social work practitioners are required to support an increasing range of learners, trainees, apprentices and pre-registration students engaging in practice-based and work-based learning within workplace settings characterised by super-complexity and constant change. This handbook aims to prepare healthcare professionals, therapists, social workers and final year students to understand the nature of practice education within a range of clinical, therapeutic, professional practice settings.

Health and social work students are increasingly offered opportunities to engage in peer-assisted practice learning where they are developing coaching skills to support the learning of junior students. Additionally, the practice of supervising and supporting students is now becoming a feature of health and social work programmes to ensure that students become 'practice supervisor ready' at the point of graduation.

A wide range of academics, educators and practice staff have contributed to the book to ensure that practice supervisors, assessors, educators, facilitators and learning environment leads are provided with a range of innovative, creative and alternative approaches to promote safe, effective, inclusive and transformational practice education experiences.

Structure

Each chapter starts with an introduction that has been written to provide the reader with an overview of the key features and demonstrate how the learning outcomes will be met. A range of activities have been designed to ensure that the reader can apply ideas, concepts and theories to their role, practice and workplace setting. Additionally, findings from research have been drawn upon to ensure that the learner voice is central to the creation of compassionate practice learning environments and the development of innovative, inclusive and alternate learning opportunities as reflected in the case studies.

Survey of chapters

Chapter 1 uses the metaphor of 'landscape' to enable the reader to make sense of contemporary practice education by identifying the key features, terrain and landmarks that practice supervisors, assessors and educators encounter, including what constitutes knowledge and the similarities and differences between practice and work-based learning. Additionally, the importance of the role of practice supervisors in promoting and enhancing learning environments is explored in addition to meeting professional standard regulatory body standards.

In Chapter 2, the role of the practice supervisor in welcoming and inducting students and apprentices is explored, including the critical importance of supporting students to identify personal learning objectives. The chapter also provides the reader with key information on apprenticeship requirements, how to adopt a facilitative rather than teacher-led approach to the supervision of learners and to support students and apprentices as they develop their professional identities and values in practice.

Chapter 3 returns to the topic of learning environments introduced in Chapter 1, by arguing that there is a strong relationship between the quality of the working and learning environment to patient, client, service user and clinical outcomes. Readers are encouraged to think about how learners experience belongingness whilst on placements and the challenge of balancing working with learning. Expansive as opposed to restrictive learning environments are explored and the reader is introduced to two models that seek to capture the dimensions of learning within health and social work settings with reference to issues such as values, culture, safety and learner identity.

Chapter 4 presents a range of coaching techniques that can be used to develop student capability within a range of workplace settings. Coaching is differentiated from mentorship prior to a survey of the professional skills needed to fulfil the role of a coach as a practice supervisor, assessor or educator. At the heart of the chapter is a comprehensive exploration of how to facilitate coaching conversations using strengths-based approaches, including the management of students who disclose sub-optimal practices.

The preparation of students, learners and apprentices for practice-based assessment is the focus of Chapter 5, with a concise discussion of the difference between formative and summative assessment strategies, proficiencies and competencies. The phenomena of students not being failed in practice by their assessors (known as 'failure to fail') is explored in the context of research findings and implications for safety when practice staff give students the 'benefit of the doubt', in addition to how to undertake a delegated assessment with the contribution of patients, clients and service users.

What constitutes a transformational learning experience is discussed in Chapter 6, which focuses on the quality and nature of learning conversations. In keeping with Chapter 4, coaching is revisited in the context of what constitutes a 'conversation that matters' but from the perspective of peer-to-peer learning where students and apprentices can support each other through guided and structured learning practice opportunities. Principles of giving effective feedback are covered in considerable detail including a range of activities that demonstrate the importance of best practice in the giving of written as well as verbal feedback and feedback that is forward-facing and future-referenced. The role of emotion is explored with reference to the impact of failing a student and a values-based model of reflection is proposed as a useful strategy to strengthen the resilience of assessors.

In Chapter 7, the attention switches to how to identify and support a student in difficulty with a range of strategies including action planning, culturally sensitive approaches to supervision and the role of the educator as a guardian of inclusive learning.

The theme of compassionate practice learning is explored with reference to quality assurance in Chapter 8, where the reader will also be able to make sense of how to work with university link lecturers and stakeholders to resolve issues arising from a dissatisfied learner. A decision-making tool is proposed to assist students and apprentices when raising and escalating a concern in practice.

Chapter 9 contains a comprehensive assessment of practice education within social work and social care settings within the United Kingdom. The nature of social work as a location of workplace learning is presented as a complex web of sometimes competing factors that present practice educators with a range of challenges and opportunities for their personal development needs. Particular attention is paid to supporting learners to engage with multi-disciplinary teams and interprofessional working.

Supporting learners working with children and young people is the focus of Chapter 10, where a range of political and social factors is explored with reference to supervision practices and the application of learning theory. The importance of students and apprentices understanding the central tenets of family-centred approaches through the development of communication skills is a key focus of the chapter.

In Chapter 11, practice supervision within the maternity setting is explored with particular reference to the nursing and midwifery proficiencies and standards relating to the support, supervision and assessment of students. Learning within community settings is also a key feature with a range of activities to support supervisors and assessors to facilitate learning within multiprofessional maternity and contemporary birthing settings.

Our consideration of community as well as secondary care settings continues in Chapter 12 with an extensive discussion of the Nursing and Midwifery Council (NMC) practice education standards and the provision of indirect supervision for learners in arms-length or long-arm practice experiences. The chapter also considers how best to supervise students caring for clients and service users with long-term or enduring health conditions prior to the opportunities afforded from international and elective placement experiences.

In Chapter 13, a range of participatory learning strategies is presented prior to a consideration of the role of practice supervisors supporting students and apprentices within mental health settings. A conversational model is explored for the development of both learners and their supervisors. Additionally, the chapter explores how to support students who challenge assessment decisions and the role of debriefing to support and develop practice assessors.

Chapter 14 provides the reader with critical information in order to support learners who require reasonable adjustments due to a range of neurodivergent conditions, to ensure that practice learning is truly inclusive. Once again, case studies are used to unpack the role and practice of supervisors, assessors and educators in upholding compassionate support for learners with diverse needs in the context of learning styles and preferences.

Facilitating and supporting learning in non-assessed, virtual and alternate environments is the focus of Chapter 15. Opportunities within the private, voluntary and independent sector are explored and include charities, secure and justice service settings, which afford students and apprentices deep, rich and meaningful practice experiences. In this chapter, care is taken to outline the need to provide a safe and supportive approach to learners with case studies that feature placements within prisons and a unique virtual experience for nursing students within primary care.

In Chapter 16, the focus shifts towards preparing experienced supervisors and educators to undertake summative assessments and transition to the role of being an assessing practice educator and practice assessor. The challenge of fulfilling a dual role as a support and assessor of students is considered in addition to findings from research that have explored the characteristics of confident ethical assessment practices. The chapter concludes with a range of activities to support transition into full-time education and academic roles and the practices necessary to transition from clinical and professional settings to an approved educational institute.

Acknowledgements

As Editor I would like to thank Dr Sally Boyle, head of School of Nursing, Midwifery and Health Education, for ensuring that I had sufficient time and support to establish the writing team and start work whilst I was employed at the University of Bedfordshire.

Professor Ann Gallagher, head of the Department of Health, has ensured that I have been fully supported to complete the writing of this book and was tremendously gracious as I recruited additional co-authors shortly after my arrival at Brunel University London.

Hollie Starbuck, lecturer in Mental Health Nursing, and Dr Michael Thomas, associate dean (Equality and Diversity), very kindly reviewed early versions of Chapter 14 and Chapter 17, respectively, and are both employed within the Department of Health Sciences at Brunel University London.

And finally, I would not be able to do anything without the sterling support of my wife, Rebecca, who like her biblical counterpart, carries her promises and helps me to receive numerous blessing.

Contributors

Claire Bunyan qualified as a midwife in 2009. She became a 'clinical practice facilitator' in 2018 and joined the University of Bedfordshire in 2020, allowing her to continue her passion for developing the midwives of the future. Claire has always had an interest in educating and supporting colleagues; after becoming a midwife, she was involved in a pilot scheme to support newly qualified midwives in their first few weeks after qualifying. Claire completed her mentorship training in 2012 and went on to have two articles published on a theme of supporting students. She completed her MSc in advanced clinical practice, midwifery, pathway in 2020. Her dissertation topic was supporting preceptor midwives to increase the amount and quality of support offered to those who are newly qualified. She encourages all students and midwives to be the 'midwife/supervisor/assessor' that they wish they had had – whether as a student or birthing person.

Dr Gillian Ferguson is a lecturer in the Faculty of Wellbeing, Education and Language Studies (WELS) at The Open University working on Social Work and Health and Social Care programmes across the United Kingdom's four nations. She has worked in a broad variety of roles including direct practice, workforce development, advisory and regulatory, as a social worker, community learning worker and academic. Gillian worked in her early career as a support worker in the Rape Crisis movement, subsequently working as a youth worker, adult learning worker and health promotion practitioner. She managed a third sector addictions counselling service for many years, remains involved in supporting learning and continues to undertake direct practice in this field. She has led the delivery of practice education programmes in social work in Scotland and remains a committed practice educator. Gillian is an educational researcher interested in professional learning and practice across disciplines.

Dr Ayana Horton Ifekoya is a lecturer in occupational therapy at Brunel University London. In this role, she has supported many students and practice placement educators. She qualified as an occupational therapist in 1997 and worked in the USA and United Kingdom in the community, acute, in-patient and outpatient rehabilitation settings with adult and paediatric patient populations including clients with amputations, spinal cord and traumatic brain injury, stroke, hip fractures and patients with complex needs arising from neurodiversity and mental illness. She completed her MBA from Wayne State University in 2002 and her PhD in 2019 from the University of Manchester with a thesis on organisational behaviour. Her area of expertise is focused on emotional labour and relationships at work.

Dr Meriel Norris is a professor of rehabilitation research and practice at Brunel University London. She qualified as a physiotherapist in 1993 and worked in the NHS for several years specialising in neurorehabilitation and finally as a clinical specialist in stroke at St Marys Hospital, London. She has also worked in India and Indonesia for a number of years in rehabilitation and developing training materials for therapists working in the community. She completed her PhD in 2009 and joined Brunel University London, where she has remained. Her previous role as BSc physiotherapy programme lead and current as programme lead for the MSc advanced clinical practice has resulted in her remaining committed to student experience. While her research interests span several areas, one is student educational experience. In this field, she has published a number of papers relating to practice and developed training tools to support inclusive practice education.

David Roberts is a practice experience manager with East London NHS Foundation Trust in Bedfordshire. He is a learning disability nurse (RNLD) and has been involved in nurse education for over 30 years, focusing predominantly on placement provision and support. He completed an MSc in professional healthcare education in 2006. Working in practice education, safeguarding, hospital liaison and in professional development, he continued his passion for improvements in education across the workforce. He has a keen interest in developing student-centred placements and the use of innovative methods of supporting nurses in their roles as educators. He enjoys exploring the use of technology to enhance professional education.

Dr Tina Salter is a senior lecturer in applied social sciences at the University of Bedfordshire. She has a professional background in youth and community work, latterly specialising in mentoring and coaching for young people. She has worked in higher education training students in childhood and youth studies since 2004 and has developed professionally validated youth work courses at undergraduate and postgraduate levels. She has experience in managing youth work placements and supporting students and supervisors to get the most out of their placement experience. She is an experienced researcher in the areas of youth work, coaching and mentoring. She has a master's in coaching and mentoring practice and her thesis looked at coaching supervision. She also has a professional doctorate in coaching and mentoring practice and her doctoral research looked at the shared and distinctive aspects of coaching and mentoring.

Kirsty Shanley has a background in finance and over 20 years of experience of working clinically within the NHS as a nurse, predominantly in primary care. Currently working in education, leadership and management, and an experienced coach, Kirsty is passionate about progression opportunities for those who wish to excel and support for those who are content in their current position. Kirsty's role as a quality lead in BLMK primary care training hub has a focus on expansion of placement opportunities for learners as well as ensuring the quality of placements. This has meant being innovative in how those opportunities are created. Kirsty works closely with practice and PCN partners to showcase opportunities and illustrate how amazing, diverse and exciting primary care is, and how learners can choose primary care as a first-choice destination from qualification.

Dr Adrienne Sharples is a principal lecturer in health and social care. She trained as a podiatrist at the University of Salford and joined the National Health Service in 1989 where she practiced for 19 years within in a variety of clinical podiatry and practice placement roles. Adrienne widened her experience in practice education when she joined a multi-disciplinary team of practice education facilitators within the east of England to work with placement providers and universities to develop the quality, quantity and diversity of practice experiences for a non-medical healthcare students. Adrienne is an experienced mixed-methods researcher with an interest in developing the 'emotional curriculum' for healthcare students. Her longitudinal mixed-methods PhD research examined the demographic and personal resource factors associated with course completion and emotional health in a cohort of pre-registration student nurses using semi-structured interviews, 'World Cafés' and a range of psychological measures.

Sherwyn Sicat is the division lead for social work at Brunel University London. Sherwyn qualified as a social worker in 2011. He has a range of practice experience from his time working in children and families social work. These include safeguarding (both as a social worker and a children protection chair), Family Partnership Model, practice education, line management (a variety of disciplines including social work students, ASYE social workers, youth justice workers, education specialists, clinical psychologists), contextual safeguarding, quality assurance and LADO (Local Authority Designated Lead) in dealing with allegations against staff and volunteers and mentoring. Sherwyn joined academia to share his knowledge and experience with students who would become the next generation of social workers and social work supervisors. Areas of interest for him are contextual safeguarding, stress in social work and interprofessional learning.

Dr Rowena Slope completed her nurse training at the University of Southampton and, once qualified, worked as an emergency nurse. She has held various clinical roles specialising in medical and nursing assessment, and pre-hospital care. Her PhD explored handover communication between pre-hospital and hospital receiving teams, and found that paramedics encountered difficulties transitioning between different emergency healthcare settings in the military and the NHS. She joined the University of Bedfordshire in 2017 as a lecturer and since 2022 has been working for Bournemouth University as a senior lecturer. Currently, she is the academic lead for the Registered Nurse Degree Apprenticeship programme and teaches on pre-registration and post-registration programmes. She has published on a range of nursing issues including handover communication, management of pressure injuries and medical sociology.

Andrea Thompson qualified as an operating department practitioner in 2002 and worked in clinical practice until 2015, when she joined the teaching team at the University of Bedfordshire. Having always been keen to mentor and coach students, the move into academia was a wonderful opportunity to focus on teaching full time. She completed her MSc in advancing healthcare practice in 2018 and is now working on her PhD, with a focus on neurodiversity within healthcare higher education. Andrea has both a professional and a personal interest in neurodivergence and reasonable adjustments, with two of her children diagnosed with a learning difference. In her professional capacity, she hopes to ensure that all learners are given the opportunity to succeed and flourish in the classroom and the practice environment. As principal lecturer and portfolio lead for the allied health professions at the University of Bedfordshire, she oversees a range of AHP programmes and this includes raising awareness of reasonable adjustments and how these can be implemented successfully.

Mel Webb is the course co-ordinator for the children and young people's nursing course at the University of Bedfordshire. Mel qualified as a children's nurse in 1995 and did her teaching and assessing ENB998 short course. She has worked on general paediatric wards and completed her oncology, nurse practitioner and V300 non-medical prescribing course. Mel loved mentoring students on the wards with their practical skills and knowledge. In 2014, Mel changed jobs and started teaching students at UoB; she enjoys seeing the students' progress to registration. Mel is very keen on developing students' skills in numeracy and drug calculations. In her spare time, Mel enjoys local amateur dramatics, gardening and patchwork.

Chapter 1

Landscape of practice learning

Mark Wareing and Adrienne Sharples

By the end of this chapter, you will be able to:

- Explain at least four features of the landscape of learning within health and social care settings.
- Discuss the workforce challenges associated with supporting a range of learners, students and apprentices.
- Describe the key factors that impact on the learner experience.
- Evaluate the role of the practice supervisor, assessor and educator in meeting professional and regulatory standards within the workplace.

Introduction

In this first chapter, we will use the metaphor of 'landscape' to make sense of the nature of practice learning within contemporary health and social care settings within the United Kingdom.

Any attempt to describe the complexity of current health and social care service provision is an extraordinarily ambitious endeavour and so we will focus on the key features that characterise what is an ever-changing and dynamic learning landscape. Learners may undertake their practice-based learning within a super-abundant range of clinical, therapeutic or local authority teams within the National Health Service (NHS) and private, voluntary and independent sectors, requiring their practice to be supervised to safeguard the learner, patient, client, service user and organisation.

Balancing the requirement for adequate supervision alongside the delivery of services may present a challenge for organisations seeking to maintain the quality of the learning experience. Similarly, the need to balance the provision of a high-quality learning environment with a productive workplace to ensure that learning and working are coincident is a key requirement of the supervision of practice that may determine the quality of the learner experience. These key result areas are mandated in current standards published by regulatory and professional bodies that describe the role and practice of the contemporary practice supervisor, assessor or educator. Professional bodies such as the Nursing and Midwifery Council, Health and Care Professions Council and College of Operating Department Practice clearly stipulate the knowledge, skills, training and preparation required of registered health and social care practitioners in their roles as supervisors of practice-based learners (NMC, 2023; HCPC, 2017, CODP, 2021).

DOI: 10.4324/9781003358602-1

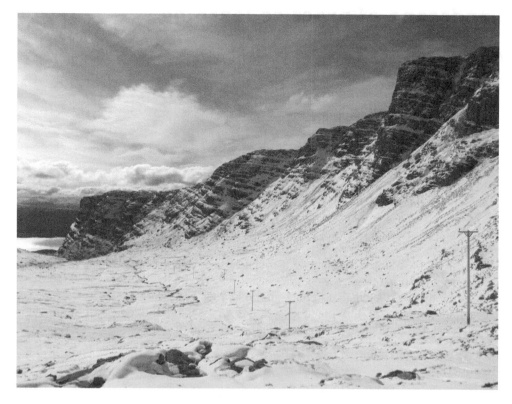

Figure 1.1 A landscape (photo taken by editor).

We will begin by making sense of the nature of practice learning as a landscape of common features that determine the range and scope of learning opportunity that create competent and knowledgeable learners.

Figure 1.1 is of the Bealach Na Ba mountain pass at Wester Ross in the Scottish Highlands. A single-track road on the left of the picture leads down to the loch at the foot of the Applecross peninsula, running parallel to a stream and line of telegraph poles.

The landscape of learning may be characterised by a challenging terrain within a sometimes hostile and changing climate in a journey overshadowed by frightening as well as thrilling features that may change our horizons.

Activity 1

Think about your experience of working with and supervising learners within your current role. Imagine you were asked to describe your workplace as a landscape:

- What would be the key features?
- What if any, boundaries exist between different practice areas?
- What pathways can learners follow?
- What fields of knowledge are available to you and your learners?

- What are the danger areas and obstacles?
- What features enable learners to traverse the landscape of practice safely and successfully?

Practice as a landscape for learning

Hopefully, the first activity will have provided you with an opportunity to visualise the terrain, landmarks and location of practice when supervising and supporting learners, including the different fields of knowledge and experience that underpin the skills needed as a successful facilitator of learning. In Chapter 3, we will engage with another geographical metaphor as we examine the nature of learning environments.

There is a temptation to visualise the role of the practice supervisor, assessor and educator in the context of the immediate team, ward or department, where the practice support is framed by the dimensions of the service provided. Thinking about landscapes of practice helps us to make sense of the wider geography of learning which traverses the workplace and employing organisation. Wenger-Trayner and Wenger-Trayner (2015) argue that communities of practice that operate within teams or departments do not represent the complexity in which professionals utilise bodies of knowledge, where different practices are characterised by history, domains of knowledge and regimes of competence. The landscape is political as professionals use particular discourses to communicate and enforce worldviews whilst complying with demands and claims to knowledge that create hierarchies. The terrain of a practice landscape can sometimes be flat, where knowledge flows from practices that produce it, to practices that receive it. Wenger-Trayner and Wenger-Trayner (2015, p. 16) describe findings from an ethnographic study where a group of hospital-based nurses were observed coming to an idea about what to do with a patient by suggesting that their idea had come from a doctor, which reflected the hierarchy of knowledge that existed within that clinical environment. In this sense, landscapes can have a diversity characterised by boundaries between practice where the history of a form of learning may not be shared with others.

Activity 2

Think about the knowledge that you use in your role and practice. Identify:

- The sources of knowledge that shape your clinical decision-making.
- The type of knowledge that has been shaped by clinical experiences.
- Knowledge that you use from training and education.

Hopefully, the last activity will have helped you to understand that knowledge is not only a resource or collection of facts, but a personal process shaped by formal and informal learning experiences that practitioners draw upon in order to practice.

Knowledgeability

Our personal experience of learning characterises our journey through the landscape, which in turn, shapes our claim to knowledgeability not only through the acquisition of knowledge, but also through how we become the person inhabiting the landscape.

Knowledgeability is defined as the extent to which wisdom can be evidenced by the possession of knowledge and our capacity to know what is required in order to practice. Wenger-Trayner and Wenger-Trayner (2015, pp. 20–21) argue that we 'find ourselves' through engagement, imagination and alignment in practice:

- Active engagement requires doing, working, talking, using and producing artefacts, debating and reflecting together.
- The use of imagination involves thinking, reflecting and using images of ourselves and others, which leads to an alignment with the immediate workplace context, to ensure that our activities are coordinated and lawful and our intentions implemented.
- The complexity of the learner's experience of the landscape, including its practice and boundaries, requires knowledgeability so that we can establish relationships with people and be recognised as a legitimate and reliable source of information and provider of a particular service.

Learning to become a practitioner requires the establishment of a meaningful identity comprising of competence and knowledgeability in a varied and dynamic landscape of relevant practices (Wenger-Trayner and Wenger-Trayner, 2015, p. 23). The role of the practice supervisor, assessor and educator in introducing the learner to the landscape of practice and guiding them through a 'boundaried' terrain requires a complex range of skills within a journey that creates the knowledgeability of both the supervisor and the learner.

Activity 3

Reflect on a particularly surprising or puzzling incident that you have had either with a patient, client, service user or learner.

Identify the types of knowledge that you drew upon in order to respond to the needs of those involved. These may be:

- Technical knowledge – relating to the use of particular equipment.
- Procedural knowledge – required to complete a procedure safely, effectively and efficiently.
- Theoretical knowledge – the underpinning rationale for providing care or responding to the needs of a patient, client, service user or learner in a particular way.
- Personal knowledge – 'know how' a technique or way of working that you have developed and that is related to the workplace or practice context.

It is possible to not only identify, but characterise, different types of knowledge used within health and social care settings that form our overall knowledgeability. Much of our knowledge is hidden and occurs when we engage in informal learning rather than in a classroom setting where learning is structured. Within clinical settings, a hidden curriculum exists in the form of norms, values and behaviours that characterise the cultural setting, in addition to the complexity, uncertainty and ambiguity inherent within medicine that requires educators to provide learners with psychological safety (Torralba et al., 2020). If informal learning settings are distinguishable from a formal learning environment, then it follows that the nature of knowledge obtainable within practice settings is equally distinct. This has consequences for the needs of all work-based and practice-based learners, who, in turn, are dependent on their educators to facilitate learning within a practice-based setting. The name of the hidden knowledge that we refer to is tacit knowledge (Matharu and Wareing, 2023). In the last activity, you were asked to identify personal knowledge that may not be formalised, codified or even written down. This practice knowledge or 'know-how' is often tacit (Polanyi, 1958) and characterises the extent to which workplaces are not only legitimate places of learning but locations where knowledge is produced.

The challenges of supporting a range of learners, students and apprentices

The development of professional knowledge within practice learning environments is strongly associated with the socialisation of the newcomer and their ability to establish relationships whilst being supported by a key member of the community. Scott and Spouse (2013) argue that the development of a trusting relationship as a befriending activity takes time and mutual openness. Practice supervisors, assessors and educators are required to gain a sense of the personal and educational background of the learner, including the pattern of previous placements that will have generated their technical and professional knowledge to date. Entry into an unfamiliar setting following a successful career, or the commencement of an apprenticeship following employment in a support worker role may weaken a learner's self-image, particularly when they are not made to feel welcomed or valued.

The identification of the motivational factors of newly recruited health and social care students provides practice partners and education staff with important information that can assist in the management of student expectations, particularly when entering practice for the first time. Asking students what motivated them to choose their career when starting a new placement, or what motivations they have to place learning at the centre of care, might be useful for educators seeking to identify and enhance students' motivation (Wareing et al., 2024). The Placement, Impact, Experience and Destination (PIED) study demonstrated that undergraduate nursing and midwifery students were more likely to choose an area of employment and continue within the profession if their workplace satisfaction and levels of belongingness were high (Newberry-Baker et al., 2023). The PIED project was established following two initial studies that highlighted the role of practice in the career choices of student nurses (Wareing et al., 2017). The influence of placements on the career destination of newly qualified nurses' experience more than doubled within the final year of study (Wareing et al., 2018), which highlighted a significant return on the investment in the support of students.

Mixed economy of learners

Practice learning environments within health and social care are increasingly charac-terised by a wide range of learners, trainees, students and apprentices at both pre-registration or undergraduate and post-registration or postgraduate levels. Identifying the range of learners within a workplace is a key responsibility of managers, supervisors, assessors and practice educators. Ideally, every worker, regardless of their role or status, should be seen as a learner in their own right regardless of whether they are undertaking a course or formal study programme. Engeström (2001) stated that learning within the workplace can be understood when the following questions are answered: who is learning, why are they learning, what do they learn and how do they learn?

Activity 4

Analyse your workplace and identify:

- Who is learning?
- Why are they learning?
- What do they learn?
- How do they learn?

The last activity will have helped you to analyse your workplace area in the context of the learning that does or at least should take place on a daily basis. Hopefully, you will have included patients, clients, service users as well as administrative, technical and support staff in your analysis. In Chapter 8, we will explore the importance of learners gaining access to the full range of learning opportunities, both within the immediate learning environment and wider practice landscape, through the use of educational audits and the creation of student welcome packs.

This mixed economy of learners requires educators and practice staff to possess a wide range of skills to support practice-based and work-based learners. A key factor determining the nature of support will be whether educators are able to distinguish between practice-based and work-based learning; two distinctly similar but different forms of practice pedagogy (see Table 1.1).

You will have noticed in Table 1.1 that work-based learners need to ensure that their learning and working are coincident, which presents considerable challenges for an employee who may have fulfilled a distinct role for many years, as there is a requirement for them to be recognised as a learner in their own right whilst fulfilling their employment contract. Additionally, assessment is not referred to in the table. Interestingly, within many healthcare professional groups the assessment documentation will be the same for both practice-based and work-based learners, although their mode of engaging with

Table 1.1 Key characteristics of practice and work-based learning (adapted from Wareing, 2016, p. 10)

Practice-based learning	Work-based learning
• Undertaken to prepare 'newcomers' to practice • Uses a range of placement experiences • A key feature of pre-registration programmes within health and social work • Professional regulatory bodies determine the proportion of time (including the minimum number of hours) that students are required to complete • Professional regulatory bodies set specific guidance regarding the role of practice supervisors, assessors and educators	• Learners are usually employees • Learners are required to balance their role as a learner, apprentice and worker • Learning occurs while working • Learning and working are coincident • A key feature of programmes such as the foundation degree or apprenticeships • Requires the support of employers and managers • May be undertaken to address workforce needs e.g. the development of nursing associate, associate practitioner, advanced clinical practitioner roles

learning within a clinical or therapeutic setting will be different based on their status as apprentices. These factors can sometimes lead to a disparity in the learner experience, both within work and when attending formal learning within the setting of a university, for example. During the COVID-19 pandemic, nursing students who happened to be apprentices were required to be deployed to work within clinical areas, whereas traditional university applicant students were given the opportunity for paid employment (Kane *et al.*, 2022), which underlined the disparity existing between practice- and work-based learners, particularly within the context of apprenticeships. The pandemic demonstrated that landscapes of learning can be dynamic, unpredictable and changing.

Key factors that impact the learner experience

So far, this chapter has described some of the geographical as well as organisational factors that influence learning within social settings. These factors may result in a collective as well as individual impact, particularly in relation to the quality of the learning environment. Fuller and Unwin (2011) have described how the nature of workplace learning practices or the pedagogy can be influenced by the organisation of work to the extent that learning may either be 'restrictive' or 'expansive'. Learners experience restrictive learning environments when there are opportunities to participate in different communities or practice by crossing job and team boundaries; where the 'host' team has a collective memory; when newcomers are given time to become part of a community and given discretion to make their own judgements and contribute to decision-making. Restrictive learning environments are characterised by learners being discouraged from crossing their immediate team or work area boundary; where the cumulative expertise of the team is not recognised; where skills are confined to key workers and managers control the workforce through targets in the absence of employees being involved in decision-making (Fuller and Unwin, 2011). The nature of learning environments will be explored more deeply in Chapter 3.

Within health and social care settings, there is a new movement to promote inclusive, compassionate clinical learning environments for all to ensure that all practice areas embrace the notion of an expansive learning environment that support the mixed economy of learners discussed earlier.

Inclusive and compassionate learning environments

The Health Education England (east of England) clinical learning environment strategy (2022) aims to ensure that patients, learners, clinical supervisors and educators are at the centre of a culture of inclusive and compassionate learning that embeds principles of inclusivity and compassion to promote the retention of students and learners. Such an approach is committed to:

- Seeking to validate learner experiences and perspectives.
- Challenge indirect and direct discrimination in the learning environment.
- Promote approaches to supporting practice learning that is co-created with learners, patients, educators and education partners to ensure that all voices are heard, including traditionally marginalised groups.

- Utilise inclusive approaches with the existing frameworks and training within supervisor and educator training and support.
- Adopt compassionate approaches to learning that seek to promote wellbeing and alleviate anxiety arising from practice experience for all those engaged in the clinical learning environment
- Remove barriers to learning and development whilst promoting retention.
- Celebrate, recognise and share best practice.

On a more practical level, the strategy recognises that learners require work schedules, breaks and access to basic resources including name badges in order to feel safe, secure and protected from excessive criticism whilst being able to raise their concerns. It is argued that learners feel accepted when friendship, team working and the giving and receiving of affection is evident, leading to autonomy and feelings of accomplishment that enhance self-esteem. Ultimately, a learner will gain a meaningful and rewarding experience when they are able to be proactive and share greater responsibility for their learning needs as their self-actualisation is realised through creative and spontaneous approaches to problem solving (HEE, 2022).

Role of the practice supervisor, assessor and educator

Professional Standard Regulatory Bodies (PSRB) have their own published guidance that stipulates the roles that can support learners within health and social care settings and are therefore key players within the landscape of practice learning.

Activity 5

Using the reference list at the end of this chapter, identify the PSRB guidance that describes your role and practice as a practice-based educator. Download the relevant guidance from the internet to answer the following questions:

1   Is your role a supporting or assessing role, or both?
2   What training and preparation requirements are required by the PSRB before you can practice and support learners?
3   What type of trainees, learners and apprentices would you be permitted to support?
4   What, if any, other roles do you need to work with in order to fulfil your requirements as an educator?

You will have noticed that PSRB guidance outlines the role and responsibilities of each practice learning supervisory and assessing role, but not learning strategies, techniques and ways of facilitating learning. All of these areas will be covered in considerable detail throughout this book, including how to meet the particular needs of learners as well as how to respond to a range of challenges when supporting learners within different clinical, therapeutic and service settings.

The Nursing and Midwifery Council (NMC) has published a range of standards for education and training covering pre-registration and post-registration nursing and midwifery education. The Standards for student supervision and assessment, known as the 'SSSA' (NMC, 2023), set out the roles and responsibilities of practice supervisors and assessors and how they must make sure that students receive high-quality learning, support and supervision during their practice placements. Additionally, the standards set out the expectations of the NMC for the learning, support and supervision of students in the practice environment, as well as setting out how students are assessed for theory and practice learning.

The Health and Care Professions Council (HCPC) standards for education and training (SETS, 2017) explain how learners can successfully complete a programme to meet the standards of proficiency for their profession and be eligible to apply to the HCPC for registration. Section 5 of the SETS (2017) establishes eight practice learning standards which include the:

- Structure, duration and range of practice-based learning;
- Support for the achievement of the learning outcomes and the standards of proficiency;
- The provider maintaining a thorough and effective system for approving and ensuring the quality of practice-based learning;
- Practice-based learning taking place in an environment that is safe and supportive for learners and service users; adequate numbers of appropriately qualified and experienced staff involved in practice-based learning.

Practice educators are also required to possess relevant knowledge, skills and experience to support safe and effective learning and undertake regular training that is appropriate to their role, learners' needs and the delivery of the learning outcomes of the programme. And learners and practice educators must have the information they need in a timely manner in order to be prepared for practice-based learning.

The College of Operating Department Practitioners Standards for Supporting Pre-Registration Operating Department Practitioner Education in Practice Placements (2021) reflects the HCPC (2017) SETS whilst adopting the role of 'practice educator' as the practitioner who supports the learners in practice placement and is responsible for . signing off summative competency and assessment documentation. Two additional roles, the practice supervisor and the lead practice educator, provide support and the overall responsibility for learners in placement respectively. Additional guidance is provided on the preparation programme for practice educators, the provision of updates, inter-professional learning and the preparation of the practice learning environment. Additionally, there are different frameworks and regulatory systems for social work and social care practice learning across the United Kingdom. While this is not the focus of this book, this is considered in Chapter 9.

Summary

In this first chapter, we have explored the nature of practice-based learning as a landscape with an exciting myriad of features that include boundaries, fields of knowledge and particular landmarks that have particular significance for learners and educators alike. We have seen that there are many types of knowledge and that over time we develop our own knowledgeability as educators, clinicians and practitioners, which is the key to how we support students, learners, trainees and apprentices. Learners as 'newcomers' need time and investment in order to feel welcome and develop a sense of belonging, which is key to their motivation and career decision-making. The way that work is organised and workers are managed is key to the extent to which a workplace is navigated as either a restrictive or expansive learning environment. Contemporary health and social care learning providers are being encouraged to adopt strategies that promote inclusivity and ensure that learning and assessment practices are compassionate as well as learner centred. The landscape of practice learning is determined by a range of professional roles designed to either supervise or assess or with respect to the role of the practice educator, both support and assess students towards the completion of either their practice-based or work-based learning. In the next chapter, we will explore the nature of facilitative learning undertaken by practice supervisors and educators in the support of a range of learners.

References

CODP (2021) *College of Operating Department Practitioners standards for supporting pre-registration operating department practitioner education*, London, College of Operating Department Practitioners. https://www.unison.org.uk/content/uploads/2021/12/CODP-Standards-for-Supporting-Pre-Registration-Operating-Department-Practitioner-Education-in-Practice-Placements-December-2021.pdf

Engeström, Y. (2001) 'Expansive Learning at Work: Toward an activity theoretical reconceptualization', *Journal of Education and Work*, 14 (1), pp. 133–156.

Fuller, A, Unwin, L (2011) 'Chapter 4 workplace learning and the organization', in Malloch, M, Cairns, L, Evans, K, O' Connor, BN (eds), *The SAGE handbook of workplace learning*. London: Sage.

HCPC (2017) Standards of education and training, London, Health & Care Professions Council. https://www.hcpc-uk.org/resources/guidance/standards-of-education-and-training-guidance/

HEE (2022) *East of England clinical learning environment strategy*, Health Education England (east of England). https://www.hee.nhs.uk/sites/default/files/documents/CLE%20Strategy%20EoE%20-%20WEB.pdf

Kane, C, Wareing, M, Rintakorpi, E (2022) 'The psychological effects of working in the NHS during a pandemic on final year nursing and midwifery students: part II', *British Journal of Nursing*, 31 (2), pp. 96–100, 10.12968/bjon.2022.31.2.96

Matharu, KS, Wareing, M (2023) 'Tacit knowledge and the role of the dental educator', *European Journal of Dental Education*, Online ahead of print, 10.1111/eje.12918

Newberry-Baker, R, Pye, S, Sharples, A, Wareing, M (2023) Experiencing belongingness on placement: A three-year cross-sectional study of nursing & midwifery students, Themed Paper, NET2023 Conference, Liverpool. https://www.advance-he.ac.uk/programmes-events/conferences/NET2023-Conference

NMC (2023) *Standards for student supervision and assessment*. London, Nursing & Midwifery Council. https://www.nmc.org.uk/standards-for-education-and-training/standards-for-student-supervision-and-assessment/

Polanyi, M (1958) *Personal Knowledge, towards a post critical philosophy*. Chicago: The University of Chicago Press.

Scott, I, Spouse, J (2013) *Practice-based learning in nursing, health and social care*. Oxford: Wiley-Blackwell.

Torralba, KD, Jose, D, Byrne, J (2020) 'Psychological safety, the hidden curriculum, and ambiguity in medicine', *Clinical Rheumatology*, 39, pp. 667–671, 10.1007/s10067-019-04889-4

Wareing, M (2016) *Becoming a learner in the workplace: A student's guide to practice-based and work-based learning in health & social care*. London: Quay Books.

Wareing, M, Taylor, R, Wilson, A, Sharples, A (2017) 'The influence of placements on adult nursing graduates' choice of first post'. *British Journal of Nursing*, 26 (4), pp. 228–233, https://www.magonlinelibrary.com/doi/abs/ 10.12968/bjon.2017.26.4.228

Wareing, M, Taylor, R, Wilson, A, Sharples, A (2018) 'Impact of clinical placements on nursing graduates' choice of first staff nurse post', *British Journal of Nursing*, 27 (20), pp. 1180–1185, https://www.researchgate.net/publication/328891896_Impact_of_clinical_placements_on_graduates'_choice_of_first_staff-nurse_post

Wareing, M, Newberry-Baker, R, Sharples, A, Pye, S (2024) 'Career motivation of 1st year nursing and midwifery students: A cross-sectional study', *International Journal of Practice Learning in Health & Social Care*, [forthcoming].

Wenger-Trayner, E, Fenton-Creevy, M, Hutchinson, S, Kubiak, C, Wenger-Trayner (2015) *Learning in landscapes of practice: Boundaries, identity and knowledgeability in practice-based learning.* London: Routledge.

Helpful resources

CSP & RCOT (2022) *Principles of practice-based learning.* London: Chartered Society of Physiotherapy and Royal College of Occupational Therapy. https://www.csp.org.uk/system/files/publication_files/Principles%20of%20Practice-based%20Learning%20CSP%20RCOT%202.pdf

Chapter 2

Practice supervision

Mark Wareing and Adrienne Sharples

By the end of this chapter, you will be able to:

1 Explain how to conduct an initial meeting with a learner.
2 Describe at least three statutory apprenticeship requirements.
3 Discuss the challenges and opportunities of transitioning to practice supervision.
4 Evaluate the application of facilitative approaches to learning.
5 Explore the role of emotion in the formation of professional identity.

Introduction

In this chapter, we will explore the key facets of the role of the practice supervisor and practice educator in the support and supervision of students, trainees and apprentices within a range of health and social care settings. The socialisation of newcomers within the clinical practice or therapeutic area is critical and requires practice supervisors and educators to ensure that the learner, trainee, student or apprentice has not only completed, but also understood the key areas contained within formal and informal induction programmes. We will explore the theoretical basis of practice supervision and support of learners with reference to the application of adult and facilitative learning theories and the impact of emotion within workplace learning environments. Additionally, we will identify the needs of apprentices with reference to the role of practice supervisors and educators in meeting statutory requirements that ensure that apprenticeship standards are met to enable the apprentice to learn and be assessed fairly and successfully.

Activity 1

Think back to when you were a trainee, student or apprentice and commenced your first placement experience:

- What thoughts, feelings and emotions did you have leading up to the start of the placement?
- How did you feel on your first day? To what extent did the staff make you feel welcome?
- What challenges did you encounter before you were able to participate in caring for patients or working with clients and service users?

DOI: 10.4324/9781003358602-2

Pre-placement student visits

Hopefully, this first activity will have brought back some positive experiences as well as vivid recollections of feelings and emotions as a student and trainee during a significant life event.

How students, learners, apprentices and trainees are welcomed into clinical and therapeutic areas is critical to ensuring that the placement or practice learning experience starts positively and is more than just ensuring that the learner feels welcomed. Where at all possible, learners should be encouraged to contact their placement area to arrange either an informal visit or hold a short online meeting or phone call with their allocated practice supervisor/educator. This is useful for the following reasons:

1 It provides an opportunity for the student and placement area to confirm that the placement has been arranged, that the student is expected and that a practice supervisor/educator and practice assessor has been allocated.
2 To confirm the start date, time and length of the placement as expected by the student and practice partner.
3 For the student to be informed of how to gain access to the placement building and who to report to on their first day and at what time.
4 For the student's duty roster or 'off-duty' to be shared with the learner so that any travel or childcare arrangements can be organised well in advance of the start date.
5 For the student to receive any pre-reading or preparatory work to complete in addition to or contained within a student welcome pack.

Additionally, an informal meeting may be an opportunity for the student to ensure that any reasonable adjustments disclosed prior to the placement are put in place in accordance with university documentation, such as a clinical practice learning agreement (see Chapter 15).

Students may undertake an informal visit to confirm their travel route or to ensure that there is safe, convenient and accessible car parking and allay any anxiety associated with visiting a new department, building or hospital site. Such an opportunity also enables the student to locate staff restaurants, cafés, rest areas, chill-out zones or places for prayer.

Initial placement meetings

Students should have an allocated and suitably prepared practice supervisor or practice educator who is assigned to work with the learner on their first day or shift. It is critically important that learners are made to feel welcome and that their identity and name are confirmed on arrival before being given the opportunity to store and secure their belongings. There are three types of induction processes that learners are required to complete:

i **Organisational induction:** this normally covers the organisational values, mission statement of the NHS Trust or employer and additional training, or the confirmation that mandatory training is completed in the areas of basic life support, manual handling, confidentiality, safeguarding (child or adult), health and safety, raising concerns, infection control and the use of information technology and governance.

Mandatory training is normally completed before the student starts their actual placement within a ward, team, department, clinical or therapeutic area.

Students allocated a placement by an approved higher education institute within the United Kingdom will not be permitted to enter practice or start their placement until they have had their occupational health (OH) assessment and disclosure, baring service (DBS) clearance successfully completed. Most universities will have panels comprising of healthcare registrants from practice partners to assess any risks associated with students who need reasonable adjustments, or any entry identified from the DBS process, which signifies a police caution, recordable or criminal offence.

ii **Local induction:** Each learner should be provided with a tour of the local department, office, team workplace, clinical, therapeutic or ward area, including where to safely store personal belongings, welfare and rest facilities, meeting and clinical/treatment and administrative areas. The procedure for summoning help in a medical emergency or cardiac arrest needs to be explained, in addition to the location of resuscitation equipment. Identification of fire alarms, exits/evacuation routes and firefighting equipment should also be included in addition to any essential service points relating to the supply of oxygen, which might need to be switched off in an emergency. Additionally, any current physical hazards or risks should be identified within the physical environment including clinical areas that are normally 'out of bounds' due to the use of high-risk equipment such clinical lasers, diagnostic radiographic equipment or cytotoxic drugs.

It is particularly important for practice supervisors/educators to ask learners what experience they have had with particular clinical observation, investigation or manual handling equipment, which may be at variance with what is used within the clinical or therapeutic area, even within the same organisation or trust, to obviate a patient safety issue.

iii **One-to-one documented induction:**

Following the successful completion of the local induction, the practice supervisor/educator needs to hold a one-to-one meeting with the student to check their knowledge and understanding of the clinical/therapeutic area and complete the induction section of the practice assessment documentation, which normally requires the signature of both parties and the date recorded of the meeting.

Activity 2

1   What is the structure or format of induction provided for learners, trainees or apprentices within your workplace, clinical or therapeutic area?
2   How might a learner, trainee or apprentice be supported to ensure that their induction is successfully completed within your area?
3   What key aspects of patient, client or service user care need to be included in the local induction of learners, trainees or apprentices that may be distinctly different from other practice areas?

Supporting students to identify learning objectives

Learners should be given the opportunity to identify their personal learning objectives within the first three to five days of the commencement of the placement or in accordance with the guidance that accompanies the practice assessment documentation. It is important for the practice supervisor/educator to examine the learner's previous practice assessment documentation or overall achievement record (OAR), to identify any documented areas of development and to get a global sense of the learner's previous clinical experiences. A useful strategy for initiating this conversation is to ask the learner about their previous employment or experience within health and social care, or other work experience and to ask them what has motivated them to choose their particular profession (Newberry-Baker *et al.*, 2023). Additionally, the practice supervisor/educator may have identified gaps within the learner's knowledge or understanding from the local induction. If the student has undertaken preparatory work and read the student welcome pack, they may have already identified some broad areas of interest that they wish to explore whilst on the placement which may relate to the following:

- Clinical care and treatment plans and patient/client management
- Patient/client/service user assessment
- Diagnostic reasoning and clinical decision-making
- Clinical and diagnostic procedures and investigations
- Communication, building therapeutic relationships
- Clinical observation, monitoring and investigation practices and equipment
- Treatment, management plans, early intervention strategies
- Therapeutic engagement, assessment, activity analysis
- Development of children, young people and parental support
- Care of the older adult, frail elderly
- Interprofessional, interdisciplinary, multi-professional working

The above list is not exhaustive. The practice supervisor/educator should also ask the student about the stage they have reached in their academic studies, so that learning objectives align with recent or current theoretical study or modular work. Learning outcomes should be written using a range of verbs (action/doing words) preceded by a statement, which clearly indicates the timeframe permitted for the student to complete the learning objective.

For example:

'By the mid-point interview, I will be able to competently perform …'
'By the completion of the placement I will be assessed proficient in …'
'By the time of my summative assessment I will have successfully completed at least … '

The use of a personal goal-setting strategy to help the student to write learning objectives that are specific, measurable, achievable, realistic and timely (SMART) may provide the learner with a transferable skill when working with patients, clients and service users to set goals associated with their care, rehabilitation and recovery.

Supporting apprentice colleagues in practice

The number of healthcare apprenticeships is growing in England. According to NHS Employers (2022), 2.9% of its workforce were employed as apprentices during the financial year 2020/2021. This percentage of the workforce had grown from 1.2% for 2017/2018, and these latest figures exceed the 2.3% target set by the government for organisations with greater than 250 employees for the period 1 April 17–31 March 2021. The variety of healthcare apprenticeships on offer has been slowly increasing. Early adopters were healthcare support workers and healthcare science associates that were approved for delivery in 2016, nursing associate and registered nurse in 2017, later followed by midwifery (2018), and during 2018–2019, a wide range of allied health professions regulated by the Health and Care Professions Council (HCPC) including occupational therapy, physiotherapy, podiatry and dietetics were approved.

The growth in the number of apprentices has implications for practice supervisors, assessors, educators and managers as there may be some employed in your team whom you are required to support, or you may receive an apprentice from another employer or part of your organisation to gain practice experience. It is important that you are acquainted with the 'apprenticeship funding rules' issued by the Department of Education (2023) as these set mandatory standards that employers and apprenticeship providers receiving funding for apprenticeships must adhere to. These standards are revised on an annual basis, and many healthcare employers employ apprenticeship leads who will be up to date in their knowledge of current requirements, so will be able to advise you of your obligations. Of key importance to all educators and managers are the mandatory requirements to:

- Allow the apprentice to attend weekly 'off the job' training. The types of learning activities included and the minimum weekly time allowance have changed over time, but it usually includes time to attend theoretical sessions delivered by the apprenticeship provider and practice experiences that may be delivered by the same provider or within a variety of placement providers. Apprentices must also be granted time to undertake their written assignments.
- Attend 'progress reviews' at least four times per a year. The aim of this meeting is to discuss the progress of the individual apprentice against their training plan. This meeting may also include discussion of any concerns, changes of circumstance that impact upon the apprentice's progress, amending the training plan in light of these issues and signing off the off the job training. While this formal meeting is led by the training provider, employers have a mandated obligation to attend meetings along with their apprentice. The meeting needs to be documented and signed by all attendees and kept for evidence in case of inspection by external bodies. Although the apprenticeship funding rules do not stipulate specific job roles that you are expected to attend, as you can see, the focus of the meetings lends themselves to individuals who work closely with the apprentice in their workplace and are involved with their progress, i.e. the apprentice's manager or practice supervisor.

While the apprenticeship training provider will support your apprentice, particularly with theory and academic assignments, it is important that your apprentice colleague also receives encouragement and assistance in the workplace to ensure that they develop satisfactorily and are able to put the theory they have learned into practice during their day-to-day role. Support that managers, practice supervisors and assessors can offer is varied and can include:

- Offering a 'buddy' who is a newly qualified apprentice of the same profession. If this is not possible within your organisation, you could try and partner your apprentice with someone from an outside organisation in the same profession, or someone within your organisation with a similar role who has personal experience of being an apprentice.
- Organising meetings and shadowing opportunities with colleagues who will play a key role for the apprentice to help them develop a working relationship and see where their role fits in with the wider organisation.
- Providing the apprentice and their colleagues with information regarding the apprentice's job role and objectives and articulating the expectation that all must respect this so that all parties are clear of what is expected of the apprentice. This is particularly important in cases where existing staff are accepted onto an apprenticeship, as many colleagues might be tempted to continue regarding them in their previous role and thus hinder their role transition.
- Providing learning opportunities in the workplace that will help develop the apprentice's skills and knowledge.
- Working closely with apprenticeship providers to ensure seamless development and support is provided.
- Raising any issues and concerns in a timely manner with the apprentice and apprenticeship provider so that the training plan can be amended as soon as possible, along with an action plan if needed.
- Performance reviews – offering regular performance reviews helps the apprentice with their development and reduces the chance of them failing to meet key developmental points in their training plan. Many healthcare apprentices will have a 'practice assessment document' provided by the apprenticeship provider where you can agree to the skills and knowledge needed within your clinical area and the timeframes that guide development and progress in performance against these. In review meetings, you can discuss how well your apprentice is doing, and agree on an action plan in cases where development might not be going as well as anticipated.
- Wellbeing – holding regular review meetings offers an opportunity for practice supervisors and assessors to get to know their apprentice better and the importance of discussing wellbeing as your apprentice might be struggling with their physical or mental health and need support and signposting to support services within your organisation. Also, note that many apprenticeship providers also have support services that apprentices can access, should they prefer.

Facilitative learning

Learning within practice-based environments is underpinned by a pedagogical approach that promotes the workplace as a legitimate site of learning in its own right, where students and trainees can not only be assessed but contribute to the generation of new knowledge. Work-based and workplace learning is closely associated with the concept of andragogy, which is the theory of adult learning. Malcolm Knowles *et al.* (2005)

argued that adults' conception of themselves develops as a result of maturity, enabling the adult to become more self-directed in their learning; that adults draw on experience when engaging in learning; that their readiness to learning helps in the accomplishment of tasks which must be personally relevant; that problem-solving strongly orientates the adult learner as it can help them to better perform in their particular roles and that internal rather external motivation drive adult learners to obtain and refine their skills. A particularly effective approach to the support of adult learners is facilitative learning, as described by Rogers (1969), where the role of the supervisor is to create a learning environment that best supports the learner to be self-directive. This learner-centred approach contrasts with traditional forms of learning based on a teacher/instructor-pupil relationship, where the expectation is for learners to receive direct formal teaching. Rogers argued that what the student did was more important than the role of the teacher as the learners' background and experience were essential to how and what was to be learned. Fundamental to effective facilitative approaches to learning is where the facilitator is able to recognise the role of ontogeny (Billett, 1998), a concept that describes the accrued variety of practice and learning experiences that creates the biography of the learner. This requires the practice supervisor/educator to identify the previous placement, practice, training and educational experiences that the student has successfully completed and to build from the known to the unknown, using a facilitative approach to support the development of the learner in a safe and effective manner.

Once a relationship has been established, the practice supervisor/educator can begin to explore how best to involve the student, learner, trainee or apprentice in the care, treatment and management of patients and service users utilising a participatory approach. Vygotsky (1978) described the zone of proximal development where an instructor sets the level of challenge for a learner based slightly above what the learner is known to be able to practice. This pedagogical approach ensures that the learner is provided with an appropriate level of challenge when introduced to an area of practice that may be new or unknown. Allied to this approach is the need for a learner to engage in learning that is scaffolded (Bruner, 1960), where the practice supervisor surrounds the learning experience with a framework, which permits participation in practice or to undertake a procedure, but under close supervision. Bruner argued that when a student is supported whilst learning a new skill, they become better able to use their newly acquired knowledge or skilfulness independently. Vygotsky's theory was based on observations of children, where it was observed that the assistance of a more knowledgeable other enabled a child to learn skills that went beyond their actual developmental level. As the student gains confidence and proficiency, the scaffold can be removed as a result of the learner being able to expand their competency, which in turn, leads to the proximity of supervision being reduced from 'close' to arm's-length or indirect. The provision of participatory learning where students are able to participate in episodes of care underpins the learning and assessment strategy of contemporary practice assessment documentation and requires the learner to demonstrate increasing levels of competency or proficiency towards a progression point, typically at the end of each academic year.

Consequently, practice supervisors and educators need to be able to identify and enable the student to access a range of learning affordances, which Billett (2001) described as opportunities within the workplace environment to engage in a range of learning activities whilst receiving direct and indirect supervisory support.

Activity 3

Think about a particularly vivid learning experience that you have had where you have been supported to learn within a workplace or practice setting:

1 What strategies were used to encourage you to be a self-directed learner and participate in episodes of care delivery, patient/client assessment and management?
2 What, if any, barriers and enablers did you experience when seeking to identify learning opportunities?
3 What learning affordances were you able to access in order to engage in learning activities?
4 To what extent did previous working and practice experiences enable you to be a more effective practice-based learner?

Practice supervision

All students and apprentices studying on professionally regulated health and social work courses are required to have a practice supervisor and assessor or practice educator in accordance with the professional standard regulatory body guidance (NMC, 2023; HCPC, 2017; CODP, 2021). It is critical that the allocation of practice supervisors, assessors and educators is completed in advance of the arrival of each student; not least, as the learner may contact the practice area to arrange an informal visit and to request their roster or off-duty.

Placement capacity

The traditional approach to the allocation of students to supervisors and educators is based on the placement capacity identified within the educational audit that will have been completed by a university to determine the numbers of students by study pathway and academic year. For example, a critical care or emergency department within an acute hospital may agree to take adult nursing and paramedic students, but may request that only second- and third-year students are placed within the department, given the acuity of the patients and service users. One of the challenges of this approach is that the placement capacity becomes fixed at the point that the educational audit is completed, which can present challenges for clinical staff during periods when there are high staff absence periods or a department is struggling to recruit new staff. Therefore, a more effective approach is when placement capacity and the allocation of students to practice supervisors, assessors and educators are aligned to the staffing establishment within each clinical or therapeutic area (NHS Employers, 2019, 2022a). The approach recognises that potential capacity exists wherever and whenever health and care services are being delivered sufficient for at least one learner to be supported during daily working hours (Borwell and Leigh, 2021). Additionally, this enables students to be allocated to staff present throughout the working day or shift leading to an equitable 'spread' of students throughout the year. We will explore the process of educational auditing, which involves the establishment of placement capacity, in Chapter 8.

Being and becoming

Two concepts that are useful in describing the experience of students as they progress through their studies ahead of registration with a professional healthcare regulatory body are being and becoming. Being a health and social work student and becoming a professional are highly emotive and complex experiences shaped by the many and varied practice learning experiences that students, learners and apprentices are exposed to during their study programmes. Hannah Arendt (1958) described labour, work and craft as a key characteristic of the human condition and regarded work as 'the labour of life' that positions human beings within the world. Being a worker and engaging in work adds to the 'worldliness' of human experience. Arendt (1958) argued that every occupation has had to prove that it is useful to society at large and that work rather than labour, authenticates human activity. Health and social care work is regarded as increasingly important to the functioning of modern societies, which increasingly face the challenge of balancing the needs of an ageing population with the concomitant demand for advances in medicine to treat long-term conditions and meet the care needs of the frail elderly. Jarvis (2009) describes the concept of 'becoming', where learning and our progress through stages of the life cycle enable us to *become* and shape our sense of self or our 'personhood'. For Jarvis (2009), 'becoming' is about lifelong learning, which is described as a type of learning that develops and transforms us through our engagement with the world so that we fulfil our human potential.

Activity 4

Read the vignette below, which features Mica, and work through the questions.

Vignette: Mica, a medical student, reflecting on his first cardiac arrest

Following a difficult day where Mica had experienced his first cardiac arrest while working alongside Fernando the Foundation Year 2 (FY2) on a ward, Mica returned home and sat down to complete his learning log, as agreed with Fernando. After a few minutes of staring at the screen of his iPad, Mica decided to describe what had happened by recalling the events that had led to Fernando and him being called to the patient, the arrival of the crash team and his observation of the cardiac arrest. The events of the day were very clear in Mica's mind and he had no difficulty describing his feelings and what went well and not so well. One of things that Mica realised when analysing the situation was how helpless he felt towards his patient. Although he felt pleased that he had been able to observe what went on during the cardiac arrest; albeit at a safe distance, Mica wondered whether there should have been something he could have done. In fact, while the patient was being resuscitated, a patient's relative had approached Mica and said, "Excuse me, doctor, is he going to be alright?" Mica felt awkward being addressed as a doctor within earshot of his colleagues and had not known how to respond. Although Mica was not able to complete his learning log, he decided to take what he had done in to work to discuss it with Fernando, as he felt he needed advice on how best to support his colleagues' other patients and relatives following a cardiac arrest.

Questions

1 What impact has this learning experience (in general) had on Mica?
2 Why might he be struggling to reflect on his experience?
3 What has he realised about his identity?

The vignette suggests that 'becoming' (in the case of Mica, becoming a doctor) is characterised by how we learn inwardly whilst fulfilling outwardly, a professional role. How learners, students and apprentices utilise activities and tools within clinical, therapeutic and working environments shape identities before patients, clients and service users as 'being' is concerned with how learning within the world leads to the development of new identities before the world. Jarvis (2009) describes how learners are given an ascribed identity prior to being exposed to a range of experiences that lead to the acquisition of knowledge and skills enabling the novice to eventually gain an 'achieved' identity. In the vignette, we saw that Mica appeared to have the identity of a doctor as perceived by one patient when in fact his professional status had been ascribed to him, ahead of graduation and professional registration when his identify would become achieved.

Values and beliefs in practice

Practice supervisors and educators fulfil an important role in supporting learners, students and apprentices to develop their professional identity. In addition to inquiring about students' motivations to care, as discussed in Chapter 1, this can be achieved by asking learners to explore their personally held values and beliefs; not least as values-based recruitment is often a feature of the interview process used by universities. Additionally, the formal assessment of professional values may feature within practice-based assessments. Cuthbert and Quallington (2008) argue that values in health and social care are moral beliefs, principles or rules of conduct that guide social interactions and human relationships. A useful activity to initiate a discussion with a student or group of learners is for a practice supervisor/educator to undertake the following exercise:

Think about the professional values and beliefs that have motivated you to choose a career within health and social care:

1 *What values and beliefs might have been **told** to you?*

- *These may be from parents, guardians, family, schooling, involvement in activity, cultural, sporting or faith groups.*

2 *What values and beliefs might have been **sold** to you?*

- *These may be from authority figures, social media, art, music, films, literature or key influencers.*

3 *As a result, what values and beliefs do you **hold**?*

- *These are values and beliefs that you regard as truth and hold within your heart or the core of your being.*

The above exercise has been designed for learners to attempt to establish the origin, roots and foundation of their personal framework of beliefs and values and to assess the extent to which their pre-existing beliefs and values conform with professional values that might be challenged when working with patients, clients, service users and relatives. Additionally, the exercise can be used as the basis of a discussion of a range of clinical situations and scenarios where students can re-contextualise their beliefs and values within clinical practice, ahead of the summative assessment of each students' professional values.

Becoming an authentic professional

Dall'Alba (2009, pp. 43–44) argues that re-shaping our assumptions about what it means to be a particular professional, such as a doctor, dentist, nurse or midwife, leads to new ways of being that involve a transformation of students, learners, trainees and apprentices. In essence, their engagement in practise, even in situations that are familiar to them, shapes how they become the healthcare professional that they wish to become, but only when they are prepared to see the everyday differently and recognise when experiences arising from the delivery of care are significant to the creation of their professionalism. As we shall see in Chapter 4, techniques arising from coaching, such as the utilising of a questioning approach that leads to 'conversations that matter', can assist learners to utilise everyday experiences as opportunities for learning and development that will help form their professional identity. This type of 'authentic' professional learning (Webster-Wright, 2010, p. 113) has the following constituents:

- **Understanding** – which leads to a change from what was previously known (the students' prior understanding) through to a transition that changes the learner's understanding as a professional. This requires the learner to know what to do, how to think and to question what is done. The exercise where students are required to identify the origin and root of their professional values and beliefs is perhaps one strategy for developing understanding.
- **Engagement** – this requires learners to be actively engaged in care and to care about specific aspects of practice while recognising that some aspects of care are uncertain.
- **Interconnection** – authentic professional learning arises from multiple experiences. In order to connect those experiences over time, learners need to harness their imagination to draw together their past, present and future and to engage with others (such as workplace practice supervisors, assessors and educators) in a dynamic way that uses shared experiences to create mutual understanding.
- **Openness** – authentic professional learning requires learners to be 'open-ended' by developing an attitude that recognises the opportunities and constraints that exist within professional environments and how tensions that arise in practice settings can be resolved.

Authentic professional learning is essential to the creation and ongoing development of authentic professional practice. Webster-Wright (2010, pp. 171–188) argues that the way a professional continues to learn is an expression of their way of being a professional in a dynamic interplay with their particular professional context. Professional authenticity arises from learning that is transformative, which will be discussed in further detail in

Chapter 6. This is achieved when learners are encouraged to seek to face up to situations by weighing-up different possibilities and seeking to understand their professional responsibilities. This requires practice supervisors and educators to support learners to engage in constant cycles of reorientation that are shaped by changing circumstances while maintaining a continuous sense of themselves as professional people.

Activity 5

Think about a recent vivid learning experience that occurred within your clinical, therapeutic or workplace setting:

1   To what extent did the learning experience alter your understanding of what it means to be a health and social care professional?
2   What impact did your level of engagement have on what was learnt from the experience?

Powerful and transformative learning experiences, particularly those that shape the health and social care professional that we aspire to be, are often characterised by situations that arouse strong emotions because of their relationship to our identity and the extent that we are personally as well as professionally invested in the work that we do.

Emotion in learning

Students face challenges during their course that may cause distress, or exacerbate mental health conditions. Some studies suggest that students experience poorer mental health than the general population, with those within health professions noted as particularly vulnerable (Lewis and Cardwell, 2019; Kotera et al., 2023). Of particular interest for practice supervisors, assessors and educators is to consider when supporting learners is the challenge some face when applying theory to practical situations. This may lead to feelings of a lack of preparedness when caring for patients, and consequently students may be worried and fearful of making mistakes (King-Okoye and Arber, 2014). Students have been found to experience empathetic distress as a result of providing direct patient care, and levels may be higher in students compared to registered colleagues (López-Pérez et al., 2013). Other causes of general distress during practice learning include experiencing ethical dilemmas with patient care, experiencing uncivil behaviour from others in placement, and experiencing heavy academic workloads whilst in practice (Suresh et al., 2013; Sasso et al., 2016; Tee et al., 2016). Inadequate preparation for the emotional aspect of practice has also been cited as a key factor in experiencing distress (King-Okoye and Arber, 2014). Stress specifically has been linked to poor academic achievement, reduced life satisfaction, feeling a reduced sense of belonging within clinical practice placements and increased health risk behaviours such as poor diet, excessive alcohol consumption and smoking (Nastaskin and Fiocco, 2015; Grobecker, 2016; Pelletier et al., 2016; Samaha and Hawi, 2016; Deasey et al., 2016). Also highlighted are the challenges faced by those who possess lower levels of personal agency. A propensity to use passive coping strategies, a reluctance to use peer support and possessing lower levels of general self-efficacy and self-esteem have all been found to be risk factors for experiencing stress and other mental health concerns (Edwards *et al.*, 2010; Priesack and Alcock, 2015; Deasey *et al.*, 2016; Goodwin *et al.*, 2016; Zhang *et al.*, 2016). There is also evidence that suggests younger students may be more vulnerable to feeling overwhelmed and stressed in practice (Galvin *et al.*, 2015). Illeris (2011, p. 20) observes that the harbouring of a negative feeling towards a person or group whose behaviour that we disapprove of can be changed when a learner gains insight into why they have acted in the way they do and signifies the relationship between cognitive reasoning and emotion within the workplace.

There are ways that practice educators can help and support their learners to develop resilience that research indicates helps individuals to manage their emotions and develop coping mechanisms.

This can include:

- Providing time and opportunity through asking open-ended questions at the end of a work session where the learner can share their experiences and emotional challenges. This is particularly important in cases where there has been a distressing incident in practice, e.g. a sudden or unexpected death or safe-guarding incident.
- Acknowledging and validating the emotions that are shared with you.
- Supporting the learner to find positive solutions through asking coaching questions to help them reframe the situation and explore different coping techniques (see Chapter 4).
- Providing an opportunity to see the positive aspects of practice by asking learners to try to consciously identify and focus on the positive aspects of their role and wider work environment, and consider things that they are grateful for at work.
- Start a 'buddy', system where senior students are paired with a junior, and provide them with opportunities to discuss their progress and any issues that have arisen.
- You might even wish to teach learners some beginner coaching techniques (e.g. TGROW – see Chapter 4) and ask them to peer coach.
- Provide ten minutes of time for learners to write a reflection on their practice at the end of a session.

Summary

This chapter has covered a large range of theoretical and conceptual perspectives that underpin the role and practice of the supervisor, assessor and educator. Practice learning starts before the arrival of a student, trainee, learner or apprentice, as we saw with regard to pre-placement meetings and informal visits. The induction process of learners is often characterised by three discreet stages, organisational, local and one-to-one meetings, where preparatory work and mandatory training need to be completed successfully before the newcomer can create, negotiate and agree learning outcomes that should provide the key focus of the practice learning experience. We saw that there were additional statutory requirements necessary for the support, supervision and progression of apprentices, whose experience of practice learning is characterised as much by being an employee as a trainee. Additionally, the requirements provide the practice supervisor/educator with an opportunity to ensure that apprentices are recognised as learners as well as workers in their own right.

The principles of adult learning were examined in the context of the role of the supervisor/educator as a facilitator of learning, who is committed to recognising the experience of being a learner, trainee, student and apprentice, ahead of becoming a proficient, competent and safe practitioner. The vignette featuring Mica illustrated the nature of ascribed, as opposed to achieved, professional identity as students practice before patients, clients and service users and we explored the impact of personally held values and beliefs and their role in becoming an authentic health and social care professional. Finally, we returned to a theme that started the chapter: the role of emotion within practice and work-based learning, which is not only present prior to, but throughout placement experiences and is central to the role of the practice supervisor, educator and assessor in promoting a compassionate practice learning environment for all.

References

Arendt, H (1958) *The human condition* (2nd ed.), Chicago: The University of Chicago Press.

Borwell, J, Leigh, J (2021) 'Addressing the practice learning and placement capacity conundrum', *British Journal of Nursing*, 30 (18), p. 1093.

Billett, S (1998) 'Ontogeny and participation in communities of practice: A socio-cognitive view of adult development', *Studies in the Education of Adults*, 30 (1), pp. 21–34.

Billett, S. (2001) 'Learning through work: Workplace affordances and individual engagement', *Journal of Workplace Learning*, 13 (5), pp. 209–214.

Bruner, JS (1960) *The process of education: A landmark in educational theory*. Cambridge, MA: Harvard University Press.

CODP (2021) 'Standards for supporting pre-registration operating department practitioner education in practice placements'. https://www.unison.org.uk/content/uploads/2021/12/CODP-Standards-for-Supporting-Pre-Registration-Operating-Department-Practitioner-Education-in-Practice-Placements-December-2021.pdf

Cuthbert, S, Quallington, J (2008) *Values for care practice*. Exeter: Reflect Press.

Dall'Alba, G (2009) *Exploring education through phenomenology*. Oxford: Wiley-Blackwell.

Deasey, D, Kable, A, Jeong, S (2016) 'Results of a national survey of Australian nurses' practice caring for older people in an emergency department', *Journal of Clinical Nursing*, 25 (19–20), pp. 3049–3057.

Department of Education (2023) *Apprenticeship funding rules: August 2023 to July 2024*. https://www.gov.uk/guidance/apprenticeship-funding-rules

Edwards, D, Burnard, P, Bennett, K, Hebden, U (2010) 'A longitudinal study of stress and self-esteem in student nurses', *Nurse Education Today*, 30 (1), pp. 78–84.

Galvin, J, Suominen, E, Morgan, C, O'Connell, EJ, Smith, AP (2015) 'Mental health nursing students' experiences of stress during training: A thematic analysis of qualitative interviews', *Journal of Psychiatric and Mental Health Nursing*, 22 (10), pp. 773–783.

Grobecker, PA (2016) 'A sense of belonging and perceived stress among baccalaureate nursing students in clinical placements', *Nurse Education Today*, 36, pp. 178–183.

HCPC (2017) *Standards of education and training, London*. Health & Care Professions Council. https://www.hcpc-uk.org/resources/standards/standards-of-education-and-training/

Illeris, K (2011) *The fundamentals of workplace learning – Understanding how people learn within working life*. London: Routledge.

Jarvis, P (2009) *Learning to be a person in society*. London: Routledge.

King-Okoye, M, Arber, A (2014) ''It stays with me': The experiences of second- and third-year student nurses when caring for patients with cancer', *European Journal of Cancer Care*, 23 (4), pp. 441–449.

Knowles, M, Holton, EF, Swanson, RA (2005) *The adult learner: The definitive classic in adult education and human resource development* (6th ed.), Burlington, MA: Elsevier.

Kotera, Y., et al. (2023) 'Comparing the mental health of healthcare students: Mental health shame and self-compassion in counselling, occupational therapy, nursing and social work students', *International Journal of Mental Health and Addiction*, pp. 1–18, 10.1007/s11469-023-01018-w

Lewis, EG, Cardwell, JM (2019) 'A comparative study of mental health and wellbeing among UK students on professional degree programmes', *Journal of Further and Higher Education*, 43(9), pp. 1226–1238, 10.1080/0309877X.2018.1471125

López-Pérez, B, Ambrona, T, Gregory, J, Stocks, E, Oceja, L (2013) 'Feeling at hospitals: Perspective-taking, empathy and personal distress among professional nurses and nursing students', *Nurse Education Today*, 33 (4), pp. 334–338, 10.1016/j.nedt.2013.01.010

Nastaskin, RS, Fiocco, AJ (2015) 'A survey of diet self-efficacy and food intake in students with high and low perceived stress', *Nutrition Journal*, 14 (1), pp. 1–8.

Newberry-Baker, R, Pye, S, Sharples, A, Wareing, M (2023) *Experiencing belongingness on placement: A three-year cross-sectional study of Nursing & Midwifery students*, NET2023 Conference, Hilton Hotel, Liverpool. https://www.advance-he.ac.uk/programmes-events/conferences/NET2023-Conference

NHS Employers (2019) *Employer approaches to building placement capacity*, NHS employers. https://allcatsrgrey.org.uk/wp/download/education/medical_education/continuing_professional_development/Building-placement-capacity.pdf

NHS Employers (2022a) *Expanding placement capacity: Ideas and approaches for expanding placement capacity for students and learners*. https://www.nhsemployers.org/articles/expanding-placement-capacity

NHS Employers (2022) 'The latest NHS apprenticeship statistics, NHS employers'. https://www.nhsemployers.org/articles/latest-nhs-apprenticeship-statistics

NMC (2023) 'Standards for student supervision and assessment'. https://www.nmc.org.uk/standards-for-education-and-training/standards-for-student-supervision-and-assessment/

Pelletier, JE, Lytle, LA, Laska, MN (2016) 'Stress, health risk behaviors, and weight status among community college students', *Health Education & Behavior*, 43 (2), pp. 139–144.

Priesack, A, Alcock, J (2015) 'Well-being and self-efficacy in a sample of undergraduate nurse students: A small survey study', *Nurse Education Today*, 35 (5), pp. e16–e20.

Rogers, C (1969) *Freedom to learn: A view of what education might become* (1st ed.). Columbus, OH: Charles Merill.

Samaha, M, Hawi, NS (2016) 'Relationships among smartphone addiction, stress, academic performance, and satisfaction with life', *Computers in Human Behavior*, 57, pp. 321–325.

Sasso, L, Bagnasco, A, Bianchi, M, Bressan, V, Carnevale, F (2016) 'Moral distress in undergraduate nursing students', *Nursing Ethics*, 23 (5), pp. 523–534.

Suresh, P, Matthews, A, Coyne, I (2013) 'Stress and stressors in the clinical environment: A comparative study of fourth-year student nurses and newly qualified general nurses in Ireland', *Journal of Clinical Nursing*, 22 (5–6), pp. 770–779.

Tee, S, Özçetin, YSU, Russell-Westhead, M (2016) 'Workplace violence experienced by nursing students: A UK survey', *Nurse Education Today*, 41, pp. 30–35.

Vygotsky, L (1978) *The mind in society: Development of higher psychological processes*. Cambridge, MA: Harvard University Press.

Webster-Wright, A (2010) *Authentic professional learning: Making a difference through learning at work*. London: Springer.

Zhang, Y, Luo, X, Che, X, Duan, W (2016) 'Protective effect of self-compassion to emotional response among students with chronic academic stress', *Frontiers in Psychology*, 7, p. 1802.

Chapter 3

Learning environments

Mark Wareing and Gillian Ferguson

By the end of this chapter, you will be able to:

1 Explain the characteristics of restrictive and expansive learning environments within health and social care.
2 Analyse the relationship between the host organisation, opportunities to promote workplace learning and learning in the flow of work.
3 Describe the context and influences on the learning environment in health and social care.

Introduction

In this chapter, we will explore the context in which practice learning takes place, namely the learning environment, which we argue should provide all learners with a broad or expansive range of opportunities. We will touch on the concept of belongingness by drawing on findings from the voices of students and their experiences of learning within a range of clinical settings. A key approach to sustaining expansive and compassionate learning environments is the support provided by the host or employing organisation who, within health and social care settings, normally employs experienced education and practice education facilitation and development teams to ensure that their employees are enabled to support and assess learners, students and apprentices. Finally, we will identify a range of strategies that leaders can deploy to promote and enhance workplace learning environments for all. The focus of this chapter will primarily be around environmental considerations rather than personal perspectives, which will be addressed in Chapter 8.

Activity 1

The following statements are from nursing and midwifery students who took part in a study (Newberry-Baker et al., 2023) into belongingness and had undertaken placements within a range of clinical environments:

'Very supportive staff that were extremely knowledgeable and helped me to develop confidence in myself' (Chris).
'The staff there were awful, not welcoming at all. I had such an awful experience there. Some nurses made students feel undervalued and didn't appear interested in our learning' (Bina).

DOI: 10.4324/9781003358602-3

'The team were welcoming and I felt that I learned a lot from this placement. The environment is busy and there was always something to do or learn. The team work hard for their patients' (Dink).

In relation to the above quotes, what would be your response if:

1 This was said by a student in your area of practice or team? How would that make you feel?
2 You had worked in an area or team (either currently or previously) that made you feel the same way – how would you manage it?

The quality of the learning environment for Chris was characterised by staff who were supportive through the sharing of their knowledge, which, in turn, developed Chris's personal confidence. Conversely, Bina was not welcomed to the clinical environment and worked with staff who did not value students or who were prepared to invest in their learning. Dink was welcomed to a placement where although staff were busy and worked hard, ensured that students had something to learn as well as do.

Making sense of the learning environment

The quality of the learning and working environment is inextricably linked to the experiences of students, learners, apprentices and trainees, as demonstrated in a range of research (Jack *et al.*, 2018; Clements *et al.*, 2016; Courtney-Pratt, 2017; Wareing *et al.*, 2018) and is known to have an impact on the outcome of practice-based assessments (Burgess and Mellis, 2015; Wongtongkam and Brewster, 2017). Over the last two decades within the United Kingdom, there have been a series of high-profile 'healthcare catastrophes' (Roberts and Ion, 2014a, 2014b), where failures in the delivery of healthcare have resulted in poor clinical outcomes as a result of patient safety errors. These have led to official inquiries that have recommended the creation of a positive learning culture (Berwick, 2013; HEE, 2016) and a commitment to clinical learning environments (Nordquist *et al.*, 2019). Therefore, the need for a learning environment that meets the needs of all practice staff, learners, trainees, apprentices and students is a pre-requisite for patient safety and safeguarding. The implications at an individual level for all practitioners are for working and learning to be coincident, which can be achieved by effective approaches to workplace learning. One of these is a commitment to 'learning in the flow of work' (Lancaster, p. 26, 2019). Defined as learning undertaken without any disruption to the work activity, this strategy requires practitioners to design and facilitate learning utilising thinking and tactics that move away from instruction to interaction characterised by the promotion of learner ownership linked to goals relevant to an individual's role and their performance. The role of the practice supervisor, assessor and educator in promoting learning in the flow of work is to support learners to help achieve those goals and monitor their performance objectively with reference to real-world data (CIPD, 2022) and insights gained from patient, client and service user case studies.

Activity 2

Think about your own clinical, therapeutic or workplace environment:

1 What 'take-home' messages regarding the quality of the learning environment have been shared by students, learners, apprentices or trainees, who have spent time in the area?
2 If you were asked to write a 'unique selling point' statement regarding the effectiveness of your learning environment, what key features and highlights would it contain?
3 To what extent is there evidence of practitioners learning in the flow of work within your area, and to what extent does this reflect the quality of the learning and working environment?

We hope that the last activity will have enabled you to build on your thoughts and reflections from Activity 1. It may be helpful to reflect again on these questions once you have explored the rest of this chapter and had a chance to consider the different components of an effective learning environment. Fuller and Unwin (2004) developed a framework based on the barriers and opportunities for learning experienced by workers in an attempt to bring pedagogical, organisational and cultural factors together that create learning environments. They argued that the development of workforces within expansive rather than restrictive learning environments leads to richer learning, particularly when factors such as the way work is organised, jobs designed, skills learnt and barriers to learning are clearly identified. The purpose of the approach is to identify features within the environment or work situation that influence the extent to which the workplace as a whole creates opportunities or barriers for workers and learners to participate in learning. Table 3.1 (Fuller & Unwin, p 130, 2004) suggests the implications of both expansive and restrictive learning environments for health and social care settings.

Table 3.1 Expansive – restrictive continuum in health and social care settings (adapted from Fuller and Unwin, p. 130, 2004)

Suggested implication	Expansive ←	Restrictive →	Suggested implication
Health and social care staff can share best practice, test evidence, make sense of new guidelines, be exposed to innovation	Participation in communities of practice inside and outside the workplace	Restricted participation in communities of practice	Health and social care staff have restricted opportunities to celebrate best practice or have their own practice challenged either directly or indirectly
Knowledge and what constitutes best practice is shared, staff appreciate other roles within the organisation	Access to learning across the organisation	Access to learning restricted to tasks, knowledge and location	Knowledge, learning and skills are restricted to the immediate service area leading to 'silo' practices and thinking
Practitioners are able to see career opportunities	Access to a range of qualifications	Little or no access to qualifications	Lack of a clear career framework, trajectory or progression that limits personal development

(Continued)

Table 3.1 (Continued)

Suggested implication	Expansive ←	Restrictive →	Suggested implication
The host organisation actively seeks to retain staff, whilst acknowledging the value of developing employees to benefit the wider health and social care economy	A vision of workplace learning that leads to career progression	A vision of workplace learning that is static and related only to the job	*Learning is solely related to the confines of the job and delivery of a defined service with little or no commitment to change or quality enhancement*
Employees feel valued and have a stake in the organisation and a stronger commitment to their department and the core role of their team	Organisational recognition and support for employees as learners	Lack of organisational recognition of and support for employees as learners	*Employees feel un-valued, disempowered and may lack any sense of loyalty to the organisation, which generates risk to patients, users, clients and the future of services*
Quality enhancement and assurance sits front and centre of health and social care delivery, staff feel enabled and empowered and client, patient, service user safety is protected	Development is used for the alignment of goals, developing individuals and capability	Development is used to tailor individual capability to organisational need	*The purpose of development and learning is purely orientated to the protection of services and the 'bottom line'. Learning is regarded in purely instrumentalist terms which diminishes personal agency and motivation*
Teams are provided with opportunities to know and understand each other and are comfortable with integrated approaches to health and social care service delivery where resources are shared	Opportunities to extend worker identity through boundary crossing	Limited opportunities to extend worker identity, little boundary crossing experienced	*The organisation, teams and departments only work with other agencies on a transactional basis with emphasis on a supply and demand model of cooperation that disadvantages patients, clients and service users and restricts choice for all*
Working and learning are coincident. There is a strong and evidence commitment to deliberately use every client, patient or service episode as an opportunity for learning including every day and novel experiences using a range of methods, strategies and artefacts	A workplace curriculum with the use of documents, symbols, language and tools accessible to trainees and apprentices	Limited workplace curriculum with patchy access to aspects to solidify practices	*A training approach pre-dominates, where learning is atomised into the acquisition of skills using a competency framework or a 'see one, do one, teach one' approach which actually embeds unsafe practice, where the values and voices of patients, clients and service users are disregarded or go unheard*

(Continued)

Table 3.1 (Continued)

Suggested implication	Expansive ←	Restrictive →	Suggested implication
Departments, wards and teams are lean and efficient as they possess skill mixes that enable a range of trainees, learners and apprentices to become proficient over and above what is required within practice assessment documentation	Widely distributed skills	Polarised distribution of skills	Trainees, learners and apprentices rely on a narrow range of practice staff who in turn, become over-burdened with supervision and assessment work
Practice staff within all departments, wards and teams are efficient and able to demonstrate significant levels of productivity sufficient for learning to occur on a daily rather than a protected basis	Technical skills valued	Technical skills taken for granted	Backlogs occur within routine care and management as a limited range of staff are able to access, enter data or maintain information management systems leading to poor service user outcomes and access issues
Staff sickness, annual and study leave causes a negligible effect on service delivery as there is sufficient flex to respond to changes in service demands and changes to patient/ service user acuity	Knowledge and skills of whole workforce developed and valued	Knowledge and skills of key workers/groups developed and valued	Practice staff lack confidence and are un-empowered leading to decisions being made by a limited range of the team who hold senior or particularly specialist roles and unmanageable workloads
An open and transparent working and learning environment exists	Teamwork valued	Rigid specialist roles	The quality of both the working and learning environment is poor
Patients, clients, service users, relatives and informal carers frequently comment on the quality of communication and staff feel valued	Cross-boundary communication encouraged	Bounded communication	Levels of satisfaction amongst service users, clients and contractors is poor leading to high levels of conflict, stress staff absence and sickness with marked lack of accountability and ownership
Managerial styles across the organisation are largely transformational within an organisation that actively fosters communities of practice	Managers as facilitators of the workforce	Managers as controllers of the workforce	Managerial styles are largely authoritarian and autocratic with little scope for bottom-up or employee initiated innovation or change

(Continued)

Table 3.1 (Continued)

Suggested implication	Expansive ←	Restrictive →	Suggested implication
A surfeit of continuous learning development opportunities, role succession planning and career advancement is evident	Chances to learn new skills/jobs	Barriers to learning new skills/jobs	Very limited opportunities for learning which is mainly training, mandatory and/or of low quality and individualistic
Change is actively and effectively encouraged and facilitated with service users at the core of change management and enhancement	Innovation important	Innovation not important	Patients, clients, service users and staff have almost no opportunity to suggest new ways of working; research and evidence is largely ignored
Expertise in addition to multiple modes of knowing is valued with each department, team or ward area actively generating new knowledge and creating and testing new ways of working	Multi-dimensional view of expertise	Top-down view of expertise	The voices and perspectives of patients, clients, service users and staff is largely ignored; only complaints operate as a locus of change

We can learn a lot about expansive and restrictive learning environments from the ideas discussed so far in this chapter. It can be difficult to think about how to maximise the opportunities for learning in any workplace setting. It is vital to understand the nature of the places and spaces that form the learning environment *and* the work or practice tasks that require to be learned. In health and social care, work is very diverse, and in some way always involves the physical, emotional and spiritual care of unique people. This means that learning in this context is very different to other workplace environments.

A holistic and integrated context model for effective learning environments in health and social care

We now introduce a holistic context model of the influences on learning environments in health and social care (Ferguson, 2021). The model weaves important influences and ingredients together, each important to consider when thinking about what it means to be learning in health and social care. We will explore the model and consider how this can help you to create effective learning environments.

People are at the heart of this model and all the different elements of context are important to consider for an optimum learning environment in health and social care. The web indicates the multiple connections and threads between the different contextual influences and essential ingredients for learning. It is important to consider all of the elements and the interplay between them, rather than a fragmented list when reflecting on a host or employing organisation. People who are using health and social care services, their diverse and individual needs are shown in bold. Practitioners are also shown centrally, to remind us of their diverse tasks, roles, motivation, personal and professional backgrounds.

It is essential to remember the individual experiences of people when developing learning opportunities and thinking about the nature of the learning environment. The individual interests, preferences and motivation of the learner are essential elements at the individual level in Illeris' (2011) model of workplace learning.

In this model (Figure 3.1), a distinction is made between social and individual levels of learning to demonstrate that there is an overlap between the working practices of the organisation and the identity of learners. Illeris (2011) argues that work and workplaces are sites of learning and knowledge transfer, but learning is seen holistically with reference to the context of the individual and their self-perceived learning needs (see Figure 3.2).

Knowledge skills and attitudes to be fostered include learners engaging in reflective activities that require them to be sufficiently motivated to seek out activities and opportunities for learning.

People who have a role in supporting learning as an assessor, supervisor, learning ally or mentor are also unique in their interests, experiences and motivation, which we explored in earlier chapters. All these individual elements meet the organisational elements when work takes place in a dynamic interchange within the workplace (Illeris, 2011). We have explored a range of organisational influences on the workplaces of health and social care, which helps us understand the complexity of what is involved in this interchange in the learning environment. We will explore some of the other contextual elements now before turning to consider who creates the learning environment and the importance of relationships in compassionate learning environments.

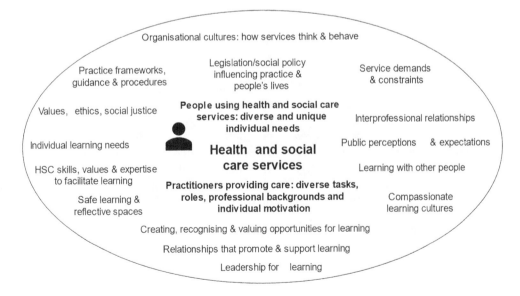

Figure 3.1 A holistic web context model for learning environments in HSC.

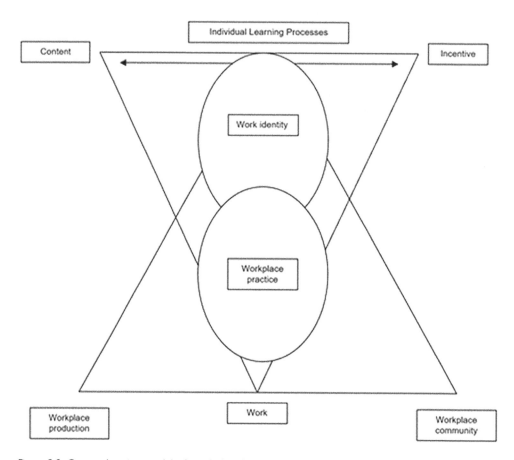

Figure 3.2 Comprehensive model of workplace learning.

The learning environment is made up of all the physical aspects of the workplace, the arrangements for working and how learning is supported on-site in practical ways. This might include provision of specific equipment or spaces that learners can use to support their sense of belonging in the team. A safe learning environment includes the physical and psychological aspects of how the setting supports the learner. We have already considered the notion of belongingness, but we will consider some other aspects of individual learner experiences, preferences and needs later in this chapter. The environment is also characterised by non-physical influences, and it is necessary to consider this context of learning. The ethos and culture of the organisation are central to the experience of learners. Organisational culture can be understood as the beliefs, values, ways of thinking and behaving. Often these become habits of how things are within a workplace and includes the attitude and value placed on learning. Culture influences how learning is promoted, supported, expansive or restrictive, as outlined earlier in Table 3.1. One of the other contextual influences on the learning environment is the legislation and social policy that influences health and social care services. Policy influences which services are funded, the shape these take, their priorities and any associated regulations, frameworks, practice guidance and procedures. This is a key aspect of learning in health and social care that must be considered in workplace learning strategies. Policy also directly influences the resources that are available for funding learning and development in health and social care.

Health and social care organisations continue to change shape and face considerable pressures and constraints, a further contextual influence on the learning environment. Delivering services while managing staff shortages, funding cuts and increasing demands provides a challenge for host organisations and learners within them. Public services face increased expectations and scrutiny at all levels. It is, however, an important part of learning in health and social care that learners understand these challenges as part of their initiation or continuing learning and development in practice settings. Learning to work within integrated settings, multi-agency partnerships, navigating communication sharing dilemmas, onward referral arrangements and working in constrained services will be just some of the expectations of practice.

Activity 3

Using either the holistic context model in Figure 3.1 or comprehensive model in Figure 3.2, determine:

1   How learning is valued and promoted in your organisation or team.
2   The wider influences on the learning environment arising from policy and guidance.
3   Whether people are at the heart of learning in your area of practice.
4   The most important ingredients of an effective learning environment.

You might have approached the final question in Activity 3 from the perspective of someone who supports learners, or from your own experience of learning. Some of the essential ingredients of an effective learning environment identified by learners across different settings often include feeling safe; being listened to; having experience acknowledged; support available; arrangements being well organised; peer support; good values and ethical approach; modelling good practice; clear information and understanding of learning requirements. These are just some of the essential ingredients. You may have identified many others that are important to you.

Empathising with the experience of learners in health and social care can help identify what will foster learning. Those supporting learning as assessors, mentors and in other roles also find themselves in the centre of a complex range of influences. Relationships between people involved in learning are probably the most important factor in an expansive learning environment. Health and social care by definition promotes wellbeing and a caring, compassionate approach. Knowledge and skills from practice in health and social care are readily transferable to learning relationships. Bridges and Fuller (2015) highlight the importance of the relational capacity of practitioners as fundamental in a compassionate learning and caring environment. This centres on the empathic ability of people in all roles and relationships in the workplace learning environment. In many ways an expansive, compassionate learning environment mirrors the skills, values and ethics of an effective health and social care service. Principles and standards of practice can be applied to how learning and development are organised and supported. We will now consider who creates the learning environment and how everyone has a role on supporting learning irrespective of their role.

Who creates the learning environment?

We have explored several ideas about learning in workplace settings and specific issues influencing health and social care contexts, but it is important to now turn to focus on who creates the learning environment. People at the individual, team, organisational and strategic sector levels all have a role in promoting, creating and sustaining learning environments. At the individual level, there are usually key people who are responsible for facilitating and/or assessing learners in health and social care. There will be different roles, depending on the learner's type of practice placement and profession or workplace role. We highlighted the importance of relationships for learning in compassionate learning environments. Relationships in the learning environment provide a supportive net for safe, reflective spaces.

Learners also have a role in contributing to the learning environment through their engagement, activities and the relationships that they develop. Peer learning is one example of where the learner might have a very clear role in fostering the learning of others. In some organisations where there is more than one learner, group or peer learning sessions are arranged. Learners also leave a legacy in workplace settings derived of their experiences. Sometimes this is in the form of induction materials for other learners, their continued involvement in supporting the learning of others or through the provision of feedback to the host or employing agency. Opportunities to harness the feedback from learners can assist organisations in their quest to create a learning culture. The learner is on a journey that integrates their personal and work lives (Billett, 2001). In health and social care there may be people with the dual role of worker and learner, in which case it is even more important to be clear about expectations, assessment and provision of appropriate opportunities.

People who use health and social care services are at the heart of the model (Figure 3.1) introduced earlier in the chapter. Many services will develop their plans in partnership with people who have lived experience to ensure that they are authentically representing their voices, interests and perspectives. It is important to remember what can only be learned in this way, rather than from classroom or indirect means. Although there has been a drive for involvement of people with lived experiences of services in education significant gaps remain (Duffy and Beresford, 2020). A primary source of workplace learning is direct practice, relationships with people using the services and the opportunities harnessed by the learner and organisation (Ferguson, 2022).

We have considered the knowledge and skills of health and social care practice as important for transferring the way we approach learners. In terms of creating a learning environment, fundamental values are also aligned. Social justice, fairness, promoting autonomy and challenging oppression are a few relevant examples that ensure an ethical approach. These values must underpin how learning environments are created in health and social care to realise any ambition of inclusivity. When difficult issues arise such as students failing assessment requirements or complaints against any parties, the emotional labour involved is intense. An ethical approach which models the values of fairness and inclusion are invaluable to mitigate the fallout of these scenarios. Prevention remains better than cure in the steps taken to create effective conditions for learning.

Activity 4

Reflect on your own role and that of others in your practice area.

1   What is your role at the individual or team level? Do you see yourself as a leader for learning?
2   Can you influence the way that learning is promoted and supported at wider levels?
3   How can you maximise the opportunities to learn and reflect on learning from lived experiences in your practice area?
4   Where are the opportunities to strengthen what you and your organisation do?

Leadership

Leadership remains high on the agenda for health and social care. Leadership for learning is seen as everyone's responsibility but the rhetoric and reality may not converge. Many individual workers do not see themselves in a leadership role but have a significant influence on how learning environments develop. The roles and motivation of the team, manager and peers are highly influential in whether learning is valued or facilitated. A leader is essentially anyone who supports, promotes and enables learning. Those involved at the frontline of practice understand the detail and nuance of the work and the environment in which it takes place. Taking a wider lens is also important for leadership, looking to the context and horizon of the practice area. Ideas about communities of practice (Lave and Wenger, 1991) highlighted the shared concerns or passions of people involved in different agendas. Closely connected with notions of learning cultures, learning organisations (Senge, 1991) and systems thinking applied to organisations Wenger-Trayner (2021) identifies systems conveners. Imagining what is possible, not restricted to own site, systems conveners think and act across boundaries to develop learning capability.

Ecology

Leadership for learning involves people at all levels and a vision for health and social care practice. Leadership is about recognising, creating and valuing opportunities for learning that have people at the heart. We have explored key influences on learning environments in health and social care, who is involved and some key ingredients. Beyond conceptions of a fixed learning environment, new thinking takes us towards ecologies (Jackson and Barnett, 2020) and ecosystems (Scharmer, 2013) for learning. These ideas help reconceptualise the systems in which learning takes place, highlighting the flexibility, fluidity and interconnected components. Within any ecosystem there is an interdependence that enables flourishing or otherwise. In very simplistic terms. wherever the opportunities lie within an individual's sphere of influence, and they act, this can hugely affect the bigger system. This is very helpful for people who feel that they do not have a leadership role in terms of status in hierarchical systems but who without doubt lead effective solutions for learning in practice.

Summary

This chapter has explored the context, influences and nature of expansive and restrictive learning environments in health and social care. People, including learners, have been shown at the heart of learning systems and relationships with others key to success. We have considered the specific issues facing health and social care services when facilitating and promoting learning. Given the pressures and demands on health and social care services, there are multiple pressures on the capacity for learning solutions that use the expertise in an optimum way that supports everyone and promotes an authentic learning culture. Leadership is nonetheless vital at senior levels with existing pressures placed on those at the frontline of practice. A shared vision of a rich ecology of learning draws in different types of learning and learners needed for the diversity of roles, professions and programmes in health and social care. Within this ecology, as in any other attention to what can make this flourish for individuals within it and the system itself, are the sustainability challenges. In the face of evolving demands, increased complexity of tasks and responsibilities in the sector, the constraints may seem overwhelming. The chapter serves as a reminder that the smallest act within the power of any individual can result in effective change in learning ecosystems.

References

Berwick, D (2013). *A promise to learn, a commitment to act: Improving the safety of patients in England*. London: Williams Lea.

Billett, S (2001). 'Learning through work: Workplace affordances and individual engagement', *Journal of Workplace Learning*, 13, (5/6), pp. 209–214.

Bridges, J, Fuller, A (2015). 'Creating learning environments for compassionate care: A programme to promote compassionate care by health and social care teams', *International Journal of Older People Nursing*, 10 (1), pp. 48–58.

Burgess, A, Mellis, C (2015). 'Feedback and assessment for clinical placements: Achieving the right balance', *Advances in Medical Education and Practice*, 6, pp. 372–381.

Clements, AJ, Kinman, G, Guppy, A (2016). 'Exploring commitment, professional identity and support for student nurses', *Nurse Education in Practice*, 16, pp. 20–26.

CIPD (2022). *Fact sheet: Learning in the flow of work*. https://www.cipd.org/uk/knowledge/factsheets/learning-factsheet/

Courtney-Pratt, H, Pich, J, Levett-Jones, T, Moxey, A (2017). '"I was yelled at, intimidated and treated unfairly": Nursing students' experiences of being bullied in clinical and academic settings', *Journal of Clinical Nursing*, 27, pp. 903–912.

Duffy, J, Beresford, P (2020). 'Critical issues in the development of service user involvement Chapter 1', in McLaughlin, H, Beresford, P, Cameron, C, Casey, H and Duffy, J (eds.), *The Routledge handbook of service user involvement in human services research and education*. London: Routledge.

Ferguson, G (2021). 'When David Bowie created Ziggy Stardust: The lived experiences of social workers learning through work', Unpublished EdD Thesis, http://oro.open.ac.uk/77930/

Ferguson, G (2022). *The importance of workplace learning for social workers*. Scotland: IRISS. Available at https://www.iriss.org.uk/resources/insights/importance-workplace-learning-social-workers (accessed 26 June 2023).

Fuller, A, Unwin, L (2004). 'Expansive learning environments: Integrating organizational and personal development. Chapter 8', in: Rainbird, H, Fuller, A and Munro, A (eds.) *Workplace learning in context*. London: Routledge.

HEE (2016). *Improving safety through education and training: Report by the Commission on Education and Training for Patient Safety*. London: Health Education England.

Illeris, K (2011). *The Fundamentals of Workplace Learning*. London: Routledge.

Jack, K, Hamshire, C, Harris, WE, Langan, M, Barrett, B, Wibberley, C (2018). '"My mentor didn't speak to me for the first four weeks": Perceived unfairness experienced by nursing students in clinical practice settings', *Journal of Clinical Nursing*, 27, pp. 929–938.

Jackson, N, Barnett, R (2020). *Ecologies for learning and practice: Emerging ideas, sightings, and possibilities*. Oxon: Routledge.

Lancaster, A. (2019). *Driving performance through learning*. London: Kogan Page.

Lave, J, Wenger, E (1991). *Situated learning: Legitimate peripheral participation*. Cambridge: Cambridge University Press.

Newberry-Baker, R, Pye, S, Sharples, A, Wareing, M (2023). Experiencing belongingness on placement: A three year cross-sectional study of Nursing & Midwifery students. Themed paper presented at NET2023, Liverpool. https://www.advance-he.ac.uk/programmes-events/conferences/NET2023-Conference

Nordquist, J, Hall, J, Caverzagie, K, Snell, L, Chan, MK, Thomas, B, Razack, S, Philibert, I (2019). 'The clinical learning environment', *Medical Teacher*, 41 (4), pp. 366–372.

Roberts, M, Ion, R (2014a). 'A critical consideration of systemic moral catastrophe in modern health care systems: A big idea from an Arendtian perspective', *Nurse Education Today*, 34, pp. 673–675.

Roberts, M, Ion, R (2014b). 'Preventing moral catastrophes in modern health care systems by facilitating the development of a Socratic ethos: A big idea from an Arendtian perspective'. *Nurse Education Today*, 34, pp. 1411–1413.

Senge, PM (1991). The fifth discipline, the art and practice of the learning organization. *Nonprofit Management Leadership*, 30, pp. 37–37. https://doi.org/10.1002/pfi.4170300510

Scharmer, C O (2013). *Leading from the emerging future: From ego-system to eco-system economies*. California: Berrett-Koehler.

Wareing, M, Taylor, R, Wilson, A, Sharples, A (2018). 'Impact of clinical placements on nursing graduates' choice of first staff nurse post', *British Journal of Nursing*, 27 (20), pp. 1180–1185.

Wenger-Trayner, E, Wenger-Trayner, B (2021). *Systems convening a crucial form of leadership for the 21st century*, Portugal, Social Learning Lab. Available at: https://www.wenger-trayner.com/wp-content/uploads/2021/09/Systems-Convening.pdf (Accessed 27 June 2023)

Wongtongkam, N, Brewster, L (2017). 'Effects of clinical placement on paramedic students' learning outcomes', *Asia Pacific Journal of Health Management*, 12 (3), pp. 24–31.

Chapter 4

Coaching to develop student capability

Adrienne Sharples and Tina Salter

By the end of this chapter, you will be able to:

1 Explain coaching and how it differs from mentoring.
2 Discuss the role of the practice supervisor/educator as coach.
3 Analyse a range of coaching tools and techniques.

Introduction to coaching and mentoring

Coaching is a conversational approach used to help others identify and work towards goals that will support them to develop or perform better. Coaching therefore provides a space for individuals – or sometimes groups – to explore aspects of their practice or learning that are important to them. A coach acts as a facilitator who helps the coachee to work out where it is they would like to get to by identifying relevant goals. Within the coaching sessions the coach will ask pertinent questions that aid the process of reflection and learning. The coach may also specialise in a particular type or style of coaching and will draw on tools or techniques associated with their preferred approach. For example, they may take a person-centred approach, or they may have specific training in areas such as neurolinguistic programming (NLP) coaching.

It is widely accepted that a coach does not necessarily have to be knowledgeable about the topic or area of practice being discussed, as the skill lies more in the art of open-ended questions, summarising, offering feedback and encouraging the coachee to think for themselves and draw their own conclusions. The challenge then can be for coaches who may have skills or knowledge in the area the coachee wants to explore, to refrain or hold back from providing all the answers or offering direct advice and guidance. Whilst there are many overlaps between coaching and mentoring, a mentor tends to have more in common with their mentee and will act as a role model and give more advice – even though mentoring is based on a conversation and goal setting is often discussed.

In many ways, mentoring students may seem more appropriate for placement supervisors, because there is a shared professional background that has led to the two people coming together in the first place. However, we suggest that taking a less directive approach by drawing on coaching skills and techniques will encourage the student to take more of a lead in their learning and development.

Before we introduce some of these coaching techniques, a word of caution. There could be a conflict of interest when a placement supervisor/educator coaches a student alongside their role in assessing practice. It is important to note potential tensions here as

DOI: 10.4324/9781003358602-4

the supervisor uses coaching to support a student to identify aspects that they would like to work on, in relation to performance, learning and development. It is important that the coach takes a position that is non-judgmental, providing space for the student to openly reflect about their current struggles and the potential barriers they may be facing that are preventing them from reaching their full potential. The placement supervisor will need to wear another hat when assessing the student, by making judgements relating to their performance. The student as coachee may reflect on an incident at work where they have done something wrong or have failed in some way. The placement supervisor will need to consider the appropriateness of re-sharing any practice-based examples discussed in coaching within the context of writing up an assessment. It is therefore important that the two 'hats' the supervisor wears when relating to the student should be openly discussed when the coaching relationship is first initiated – we will look at the coaching agreement and boundaries later.

Using coaching approaches within supervision can be particularly helpful when supporting students to grow. This is because coaching is underpinned by the belief that anyone who wants to learn and grow can transform with the right kind of support. Coaching sessions also provide focused time for the student to talk about their progress and reflect on their learning. By being shown care, attention and time, the possibilities are endless. Follow-up sessions also build on accountability where the coach can ask how things have changed or developed since the last session. So long as there is trust and rapport, the student should feel motivated to report back and start to evidence growth and transformation (Table 4.1).

Table 4.1 Key differences between coaching and mentoring

Coaching	Mentoring
Good interpersonal skills required; can be either one-to-one or group-based; both are framed around learning and development.	
More facilitative and less directive	More directive with appropriate advice
The coach does not need sector expertise	The mentor should have the knowledge and expertise the mentee is looking to gain
Usually, a short- to mid-term relationship	Usually, a longer-term relationship
Focuses on performance and is driven by goal setting	Takes place at key transitional moments and is focused on development
Predominantly formal	Can be formal, informal, or semi-formal
Coaching is not included in professional standards for practice education (e.g. NMC, 2023; HCPC, 2017). However, the practice supervisor role complements a coaching approach, and coaching has been introduced at a local level by practice providers and associated training institutions. The coaching role can also be undertaken by a fellow student.	Mentors and mentoring were previously associated with professional standards of practice supervision and assessment in nursing, midwifery and some other health professions (e.g. NMC, 2008). The mentor was a registrant who had undertaken training that met the regulator's standards and acted as a supervisor and assessor of practice.

(Continued)

Table 4.1 (Continued)

Coaching	Mentoring
Coaching relationships start with a written agreement between the coach and coachee where mutually agreed principles covering the length and number of sessions, confidentiality, professional responsibilities, record keeping and boundaries are included.	Mentoring relationships might not mutually agree timeframes and professional responsibilities if they fall outside relationships required by professional standards.

Activity 1

Carry out your own coaching and mentoring self-assessment on the ways in which you support others professionally in their development, using the following questions:

- How much coaching and/or mentoring features in your interactions – either formally or informally – and how do you decide when to take which approach?
- Is it something you are consciously aware of?
- How might you be more thoughtful and strategic in your coaching and mentoring interventions?

Placement supervisor as coach

Here we outline the key skills needed as a coach, both personally and professionally, and consider different elements of the coaching relationship and processes which might be useful to a placement supervisor.

Personal skills needed to coach and setting a coaching environment

As outlined above, coaching usually takes place for a focused period of time and therefore a key skill of coaches is to be able to draw on interpersonal skills to enable them to connect and build rapport quickly. These include listening, asking intelligent questions and working holistically to best understand the coachees' context and current challenges. A common theme that coaches often explore is helping coachees become more confident in their professional role and to work on areas to increase performance. Therefore, it is crucial that coaches can help identify areas that would best help the coachee to learn and grow. Some coaches assess these needs formally – others use conversation and dialogue to help establish the purpose of the coaching. It may be helpful to develop a referral form or invite the coachee to complete a self-assessment either in advance of the coaching, or during the first session, to help establish why and how you are going to work together. This does require the coach to have self-knowledge and the ability to articulate to the coachee what they bring to the relationship as a coach and how they intend to work. This will also set the tone of how formal or informal these coaching sessions are going to be. Coaching as a health or social care professional differs to other types of coaching in that you must always be aware of the relevant professional regulatory standard body requirements including your professions' code, standards of training and the behaviours expected within your profession or organisation.

A key skill of coaches is to develop the art of asking 'clever questions' (Rogers, 2008). This relies on the coach to put aside their own experiences and biases and ask the coachee open-ended, non-biased questions, to allow the coachee to think the question through completely from their own experience. The coach may not know before a question is posed if this is going to be the part of the conversation, where the coachee discovers a key new insight about themselves. Part of the joy of coaching is to observe the coachee go on a journey of self-discovery, whilst the coach 'holds their hand', witnessing them start to gain fresh insights about themselves. This in turn gives the coachee the impetus and confidence to try new things.

The range of key skills that are important in practice as a health or social care professional can be grouped under the following headings.

Professional skills

- *Maintain confidentiality:* You must always keep the content of your coaching sessions confidential except in cases where patient/service user safety is in danger, or a fitness to practice issue has been disclosed. It is good practice to keep a brief record of your coaching session in a meeting report form (see Table 4.2). As sessions progress you can reflect on your coachees' development and the coachee will also have a record of their actions to complete before the next session. Store any coaching documentation in a safe place with secure access, adhering to local record-keeping procedures.
- *Be professional and reliable:* Conduct your coaching practice in a professional manner. Ensure that you turn up promptly for sessions, book a room where sessions

Table 4.2 Coaching agreement form

Coaching agreement

Name of coachee:

Name of coach:

This agreement is designed to encourage you both to think about what you expect from the coaching and what you will give to the relationship. It is up to you both to discuss and negotiate basic rules as to how you will manage your relationship. You can write as much or as little as you like. Some suggested prompts are listed below as guidelines but you may think of others.

The aims of the coaching:

Time – how often will you meet and punctuality:

Attitudes toward each other:

Boundaries for the relationship:

Confidentiality:

Other

| **Signatures:** | **Coachee** .... | **Date** .... |
| | **Coach** .... | **Date** .... |

can be held without others overhearing and without disruption. Ensure that you are trustworthy and do not disclose to others the content of your coaching conversations.

- *Exhibit emotional intelligence:* This is the ability to be self-aware by recognising your own feelings and those of others. This is essential during coaching sessions as you must suspend value judgements and manage your own emotions, be empathetic to the coachee's feelings about their issue and ability to develop.
- *Be reflective:* Health and social care professionals need to reflect upon their professional practice (NMC, 2019). Those who coach are also required to reflect and develop insight into their areas of strength and development as a coach and the effectiveness of the sessions that they are involved in terms of motivating and prompting action for change in the coachee.

Interpersonal skills

- *Build rapport:* You can achieve rapport by showing a warm and welcoming demeanour and genuine interest in your coachee. Create a comfortable atmosphere by ensuring that you use the coachee's name, are positive in vocal tone, make eye contact, smile, use their name where appropriate. In subsequent sessions you can recap the previous session's content and check the coachee has followed up on their actions so that the present session can build upon previous discussion. The meeting report form will help you with this.
- *Be open-minded:* As a coach, you will be working with others from different personal and professional backgrounds. It is important to be able to respond constructively to them and find solutions to issues that you have not considered before as they may think and behave differently to you. Finding out about your coaches' background at the start of the coaching is helpful in building rapport. You might wish to ask how they think their background might impact their coaching engagement and progress and ask for feedback at the end of each session so that you can tailor your practice to their individual needs.
- *Provide challenge and motivation:* A main aim of coaching is performance development. While supportive feedback is useful, the ability to ask questions to challenge self-limiting beliefs, prejudices and encourage exploration of options the coachee has not previously considered is necessary to change unhelpful mindsets and behaviours that have previously yielded poorer outcomes.

Communication skills

- *Active listening and observation:* Actively listening without interruption and showing patience during the session will help you gain an understanding of the coaches' perspective. By also observing their body language, you hear both the spoken words and the underlying message that they are trying to share with you.
- *Questioning:* The ability to ask open-ended questions and probe where necessary to examine the deeper meaning of what is being said offers the opportunity for the coachee to reflect, self-assess and explore issues in more depth.
- *Offering feedback on practice progression:* Listen to the coaches' view on their progress without interruption. Where possible, paraphrase back to them to allow the coachee to reflect on what they have shared with you. By asking carefully chosen

open-ended probing questions, the coachee may provide their own insight on how they are progressing and decide on the best course of action to develop their practice without you offering direct feedback and solutions. Where you are required to give feedback on practice development or where the coachee asks you to offer suggestions for a solution to an issue, it is important in your role as a coach that you do so in a way that promotes self-worth, self-confidence and motivation. Be aware that your tone of voice can impact on how the message is perceived, and ensure the content of your message is clear, simple and concise. Help the coachee to set their own growth-orientated goals that conform to the SMART framework: Specific, Measurable, Achievable, Realistic and Time-bound.

The coaching agreement and meeting report forms

As has already been intimated, it is important that the coaching tone is set from the outset as this will help reassure the coachee that the coaching sessions are to be a treasured space where the coachee can openly talk about their triumphs, hopes and fears. The coaching agreement should take place in the first coaching session, which is a facilitated conversation led by the coach exploring the boundaries of the relationship. These can be negotiable, but it is important that the coach goes into this first session clear about their own boundaries. Within health and social care professions, it is important that you are up to date with your professional regulatory standard body code and standards and are clear to the coachee (student) that if they disclose a patient/client safety or safeguarding concern, you have a duty to act upon the disclosure.

Typically, the agreement should include some practical information about where and when the sessions will take place including frequency and coach availability outside of coached sessions. There may be other boundaries you both want to explore, such as modes of contact – should you give out your personal mobile number, for example? It may be that a third party should also be part of the agreement if there is another person with oversight of the coaching. It is always good practice to have the contents of the agreement written down, even if this is put in writing in an email. Agreements can always be revisited if a situation arises that causes you or the coachee to identify something that was previously missed out, so do make this point when the agreement is first drawn up so the coachee is aware that the agreement can be revisited.

Facilitating conversations using coaching techniques

The ability of the coach in being able to listen to the coachee and then ask probing, meaningful questions that allows the exploration of different solutions is a key coaching skill. It can sometimes be challenging for those new to coaching to lean more towards posing questions rather than helping or advising around goal-setting or suggesting solutions to problems. Similarly, it can also be challenging for students new to coaching if they have expectations that the coach is going to offer more guidance and direct advice. However, it is important to set the 'coaching tone' right from the outset, as this will benefit the coachee in the longer run.

Input into the coaching discussion should be limited. Aguilar (2017) suggests that the amount of talking a coach does should be somewhere between 10 and 33% of a coaching session. Remembering this division helps coaches to limit their input and keep the focus on the coachee. When coaches first start their practice, it is helpful to have a list of coaching questions to help guide the conversation. As coaches gain more experience, they will learn to adapt questions and develop their own coaching style. Printing a coaching model such as the TGROW model depicted in Figure 4.2 out on paper, for use in the coaching session that the new coach can work through is also useful and can serve as a useful aid de memoire.

Getting the coaching conversation started

Starting a coaching conversation can be difficult. A simple *'what do you want to achieve from this coaching session?'* or *'what issue from practice would you like to discuss today?'* can start the conversation. But coaches often have many things they would like to discuss at one time. If this occurs, the coach can ask them to pick the three which are of greatest importance.

'You seem to have a few issues concerning your professional practice that you would like to discuss today, which are you top three areas that you would you like to focus on?'

From here, the coach can ask the coachee to rank in order of priority the issues and start with the most pressing. Often, individuals find that if they can find a solution to this, more minor issues are resolved in turn.

Open-ended questions

Try and avoid questions that can be answered with a simple yes or no as this will limit reflection and exploration of the matter in hand. Questions that begin with where, who, what, how and when are more useful and aid a reflective conversation. The use of 'why' questions need careful consideration as they can be perceived as judgemental or critical and can hinder the coaching relationship. Here are some examples of open-ended questions:

- What challenges are you experiencing in your placement now?
- What result are you trying to achieve?
- When do you think you can practice this skill?
- How have you already taken any steps towards achieving this skill?

Reflective questions

Coaching conversations should encourage reflection to allow the coachee to move from their subjective experience to one where they can distance themselves and take a more objective perspective. By asking reflective questions, the coach can encourage the coachee to look at an issue from new angles. This can result in the coachee considering a wider range of options available to them. It is important that the reflective questions asked are 'value-free' and encourage the coachee to gain a better insight into own performance or behaviours without fear of judgement.

- What is the first step you need to take to achieve your goal? How can you achieve this?

- What challenges do you think you might encounter? How could you best tackle them?
- What would happen if you did that?
- What advice would you give to a fellow colleague facing a comparable situation?
- How will you know when you have achieved your goal?
- What are three actions you can achieve this week?

Scoring questions

It can be useful for coaches to ask scoring questions to rate a situation out of ten as the strength of the response demonstrates the current position of the coachee and can open a conversation on ways to increase or decrease the number as appropriate.

- On a scale of one to ten, how concerned are you about this situation? What actions could you take to lower this score?
- On a scale of one to ten, what is the likelihood of your plan succeeding? What would it take to make it a ten?
- On a scale of one to ten, how committed/motivated are you to doing it? How can you increase this?

Resisting the temptation to micro-manage

It is not unusual for coaches who have an assessment role to have a shared professional background to the coachee. Therefore, there is a very strong pull for the coach to draw on – and share with the coachee – their own professional experiences to help either demonstrate knowledge and understanding, empathy or offer practical help and guidance. Alternatively, the coach may instinctively know that the way in which a coachee is handling or considering a specific professional situation is simply wrong! This poses some questions for coaches to consider before they wade in and offer advice and guidance. Will telling or instructing the coachee support them in their learning and development? It may well be that some direct guidance is needed, certainly if there are patient safety or safeguarding issues at stake. However, it may be that for some coaches in less serious situations, they need to be able to explore that learning for themselves and the experiential process itself will have a more powerful impact than simply being told or advised on what to do. Therefore, the coach needs to be constantly self-reflecting in the moment, evaluating what they are saying and how they are saying it, to always ensure the best outcomes for the coachee, no matter how frustrating it may be at times to 'bite your tongue.'

Facilitating learning using a strengths-based approach

Coaching programmes are established for different reasons, but often there is an underlying belief that those being coached need help and support and are therefore lacking in some way. As we've already mentioned, coaching places an emphasis on performance and when a student is in training, the assumption is that they have a lot to learn. However, many students bring with them past experiences and knowledge that are hugely valuable and often transferable to their current professional context. This is where a strengths-based approach acknowledges those assets and supports the coachee to think about where and how they might apply their strengths to any current challenges they may be facing, either professionally or personally. Linley and Harrington (2006) posit that a strengths-based coach approach helps harness the coachees' performance potential because the focus on what they already know or are good at helps increase engagement, energises discussions and motivates them in the pursuit of their goals. When the coach has a good understanding of this, their facilitation and questions will be orientated around exploring what is already known, experienced or where the coachee has already demonstrated excellence or ability. Once these assets have been uncovered the discussion can turn to how they might be recontextualized to new or unknown areas, helping provide the coachee with confidence to move forward.

How to follow up when students disclose sub-optimal practice in a coaching session

Here are some suggestions and tips of what to do if a student discloses anything about their practice that may set some alarm bells ringing:

- In professional practice, it is important that you are familiar with and follow the guidance on professional duty of candour (see NMC/GMC, 2022 duty of candour guidance) and any associated local policies.
- If a disclosure is made within a coaching session of an adverse incident or near miss that may have led to a person being harmed or where sub-optimal care was provided it is important to provide a non-judgemental response.
- You may also need to inform a link lecturer/tutor from the student's educational establishment where the issue can be reported in keeping with organisational requirements.
- Depending on the incident, the student may need a psychological debriefing session before practice developmental work can be undertaken.
- When suitable to do so, a mutually agreed development plan can be devised. It is important to again emphasise that you value the student's honesty, and the discussion in the coaching session is an educational opportunity to reflect on the issue and develop practice rather than a formal performance management discussion.
- A coaching approach may be suitable to facilitate a conversation led by the student to describe their performance, explain why they think it was sub-optimal and explore developmental strategies to formulate a plan.
- Other options may be to take an appreciative enquiry or motivational interviewing approach.
- Always follow your professional regulatory body standards, code and local policies.

Coaching models

In this section, we introduce two models that can be used within a coaching conversation. At first, you may feel more confident to print out the model and stick to it closely. However, as you gain competence and confidence, you will find your own voice as a coach and will be able to tweak models to suit your personal coaching style and adapt to the coachees' need in that individual session.

TGROW

The first model is TGROW, which was adapted from the GROW model (Downey, 2003). The TGROW model is commonly used in coaching practice (see Figure 4.1), and a model suitable for those new to coaching practice.

This model is easy to use and offers a step-by-step process to support the coachee to identify something they would like to work on and explore potential options available to them.

- Topic – This step starts the coaching conversation and helps identify the coachee's current priorities. An example of a question at this stage might be: *'What is your main issue from practice that you would you like to discuss today?'*
- Goal – Here the conversation turns to goal setting. This might be immediate goals, or longer term if appropriate. *'What is your aim? What would you like to achieve in the short/ medium/ long term?'*
- Reality – This section of the coaching conversation provides an opportunity for the coachee to assess their current situation in relation to their goal. *'Where are you in relation to your goal?' 'What stops you from moving forward?' 'What needs to change?'*
- Options – Building on the previous section, questions that allow the coachee to explore different options and their consequences in the current situation or future. Remember, the purpose of coaching is to allow individuals to take a new perspective and it is important that you as the coach facilitate the coachee to explore ways forward

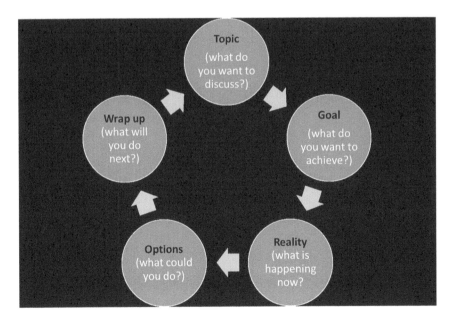

Figure 4.1 The TGROW model.

that they might not have considered before. Questions may include: *'What would be the best outcome? What are the first steps do you need to take?' 'Think of a trusted person in your life. What might they suggest?' 'What opportunities are there to think of a creative, novel alternative solution?'*

- **Wrap Up** – In this closing section, you will support the coachee to sum up what they have taken from the session and what their immediate next steps will be. This will provide a good starting point for the next coaching session to follow up on any initial steps and specific actions that were agreed on. *'What will be your next steps?' 'When will you take these first steps?' 'What will you have achieved by our next session?'*

Kolb's reflective model

The second coaching tool might be familiar to those working in healthcare as it can be used as a reflective model. There are some overlaps with the TGROW model. However, Kolb's (1984) model helps underline and emphasise the importance of reflective practice. The model will also give the coachee an early experience of seeing how reflective practice can be used within the context of continual professional development. Reflection in professional practice allows individuals to process an event in a systematic way to learn from it. David Kolb's reflective experiential learning cycle (1984) is a framework often used in health and social care and seen by many as a key tool for continuous professional learning and practice development.

Kolb (1984) describes four key stages that individuals move through. Below we suggest how a coach could use this cycle as a way of helping to facilitate a conversation, particularly where a reflective approach might be helpful in providing space for the coachee to give some deeper thought into a particular issue or area of practice.

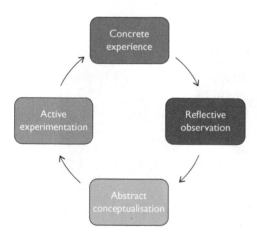

Figure 4.2 Kolb's reflective model (1984).

Concrete experience

Within a coaching session, the process of learning from reflection starts with recalling a first-hand experience. It is therefore important that the coachee is helped to identify a situation that they want to learn from in order to grow professionally. Here, coaches can use open questions to identify a key priority and obtain a description of the experience, feelings, and thoughts at the time (see also section D on getting the coaching conversation started and using open and reflective questions).

Reflective observation

The skill of the coach is to facilitate the coachee to distance themselves from their practice experience so that it can be considered more deeply. Here, the coaching discussion needs to focus on reviewing the effectiveness of the practice situation, actions taken at that time and evaluate what has been learnt to inform future professional practice.

In this second stage, the emphasis is on the coachees' experience and links to their professional knowledge, skills, and emotions during the practice situation. As a coach, you can check your understanding of the situation by using several techniques, such as reflecting back the coachees' words verbatim, paraphrasing the coachees' words or giving choice '*I think you said* ...., *these are my words* ..., *to summarise* ...'

Sometimes recalling a particularly difficult practice experience will evoke a strong emotional reaction. It is important to acknowledge the coachees' feelings and the use of 'what' questions can help: '*What are you feeling right now?*' '*What emotions are you comfortable about exploring in this session?*'

Abstract conceptualisation

Here, the coach asks questions that facilitate the coachee to make sense of their experience including questions to explore why it went the way it did, what the experience means to the coachee and imagine different ways to develop and improve. At this stage, the coach can introduce some more theoretical concepts to help the coachee gain further insight. One way to do this is by posing a hypothesis. Firstly, 'agreement' with your coachee: '*I have a theory about this situation – can I share this with you?*' Provide a 'hypothesis': '*I believe what might have occurred is* ... .' Finally, check for validity of your hypothesis: '*What are your thoughts on that?*' '*What elements of truth can you find in that?*'

Another technique if the coachee is 'stuck' in generating suggestions for growth is the 'empty chair' technique, a key concept taken from Gestalt therapy (Perls *et al.*, 1951) that allows the coachee to look at a situation from another perspective to gain insight. Here, the coachee sits across an empty chair to explain their situation to a person of their choice. Within clinical practice this may be a trusted individual with the necessary skills and knowledge needed to support the coachee in their practice development. Once the coachee has finished explaining their situation, they sit in the empty chair to respond from the other person's perspective. Changing seats can be repeated as often as needed until the coachee has gathered some ways in which they can move forwards.

Active experimentation

The coaching session ends with this final stage, where a plan of how to do things differently and goal setting occurs. The coachee should also be provided with an opportunity to explore alternative outcomes and how things might be after actions are taken. A meeting record form can be used to document agreed goals and next actions. Some of these will work, while others will be less successful. Nonetheless, testing different ideas for practice development will provide concrete experiences that can be explored in future coaching sessions (Table 4.3).

Table 4.3 Examples of questions for coaching session underpinned by Kolb's (1984) reflective model

Stage of Kolb	Examples of questions
Concrete Experience	• What issue from practice would you like to discuss today, and what are the key aspects of your experience you want to discuss and learn from in this session? • What is your goal from today's coaching session? • What could we discuss that would have the most impact on your practice development? • What happened and what factors contributed to the situation? • What are your reasons for wanting to explore this topic? • How were you feeling at the time? • What were you feeling?
Reflective Observation	• Describe the aspects of your care that worked in this situation. • What aspects could you improve upon? • Why did the situation arise? • What aspects of your practice can you develop to improve patient outcomes and experience in a similar situation? • What have you learned from this situation?
Abstract Conceptualisation	• What strategies worked well in the past? • What would happen if you did nothing? • What would be alternative options? • How would you like things to be? • What can you do that is in your control to move the situation forwards? • What do you think a trusted, suitably experienced colleague might do in a comparable situation? • What literature can you consult to get a better understanding and further ideas?
Active Experimentation	• Explain your next steps to me. • What are the first actions to take? • How will you know if you have been successful? • What will happen once you achieve your goal? • On a scale of 1–10, how confident are you with achieving your actions? • Who has the expertise to support you? • When should we meet again?

Here is an example of how reflection can be used within coaching to enable a learner to resolve a communication difficulty:

Vignette of a coaching session

During a coaching session, Tamara explained to her coach that she was finding it difficult getting hold of a colleague whom she had been asked to work closely with whilst on placement. This colleague didn't not seem to be readily available and was not responding to emails. This was particularly frustrating as Tamara's mid-point assessment was due in a few weeks and she urgently needed to get feedback from the colleague to progress with her studies. Her coach, Macayla, suggested they look at the Kolb reflective cycle as a way of exploring the issue and identifying a solution. Macayla started to ask questions about the experience to try and identify whether the unavailability of the colleague was a new thing or if this had been consistent with previous encounters. Tamara said that it seemed relatively new as the colleague had met her on several occasions when the placement first started and had also been good at responding to emails. From these discussions, Tamara reflected that she had been feeling ignored and overlooked, which she had started to take personally, which in turn had affected her motivation at work. Tamara considered ways in which she might be remotivated to try other forms of communication and not give up on her colleague, the more she considered how supportive they had previously been at the outset. Together, Tamara and Macayla thought of new ways for Tamara to approach her colleague, including attending a work event that week so she could try and get have a face-to-face conversation with the colleague, pressing the need for them to meet up soon. As a result of the coaching session, Tamara left feeling confident that she had a plan of action and more motivated to continue giving her studies and placement her all.

Activity 2

Look for an opportunity to try out the TGROW and Kolb's (1984) model in your practice. Write some reflective notes on how these sessions went and how you might further utilise these models in your future practice.

Developing a coaching culture in the workplace

Using a coach approach within the workplace will always be more effective if it sits within a wider 'coaching culture' across the organisation. Coaching conversations provide others with the opportunity to reflect and grow and lead to transformational change, both for individuals, teams and organizations.

Many organisations are now more aware than ever about the need to help create supportive working environments which encourage employees to embrace lifelong learning. Over the past two decades there has been growing interest in positive psychology to develop the growth-orientated personal resources seen in the many individuals who are flourishing (see Seligman and Csikszentmihalyi, 2000 for an introduction). Positive approaches build on a belief that all individuals possess an innate capacity for growth and self-actualisation. Key personal resources such as psychological capital (comprising of resilience, self-efficacy, hope and optimism), reflective ability and emotional intelligence can be developed with appropriately focused interventions.

Health and social care professionals report higher levels of personal resources, such as resilience, optimism, hope and self-efficacy, collectively known as 'psychological capital' (Luthans and Avolio, 2014). These have been found to report a range of positive job-related outcomes including high role performance, job satisfaction, better mental health and lower turnover intent (e.g. Sun *et al.*, 2012; Pisanti et al., 2015; Dwyer *et al.*, 2019; Hasson *et al.*, 2021; Ho and Chan 2022). Coaching is of importance as is one approach that can contribute either directly or indirectly towards the growth of personal resources and associated positive outcomes within professional practice (Grant and Kinman, 2014; Yusuf *et al.*, 2018; Hurley *et al.*, 2020).

Developing coaching communities of practice

Communities of practice (CoP) are groups of people who share an interest and through regular social interaction develop their skills and knowledge (Wenger-Trayner, 2015). Within health and social care, these can often be formal interest groups with invited members who have specific professional skills and knowledge, or informal networks of likeminded people that can develop over time within practice settings such as a hospital ward or a community clinic.

Research indicates that coaching relationships offer many benefits including helping develop stress management skills, enhancing personal development and fostering social support, a key resource for resilience building and emotional wellbeing. Added to which, CoPs also promote feelings of belonging, the sharing of expertise and support with problem solving (Wenger *et al.*, 2002).

By sharing your interest and enthusiasm of coaching with your colleagues, a CoP network can develop within your workplace to the mutual satisfaction of all.

- *If you are interested in setting up a coaching network, perhaps advertise through channels within your workplace to identify who has expertise in coaching, and others who want to learn how to coach.*
- *Finding a senior leader within your organisation to act as a 'sponsor' is also helpful. They might be able to support additional coaching training and access to other resources such as allowing time to organise events and access rooms, that can help get your CoP off the ground and sustain the network. Be clear about selling the benefits that you anticipate a coaching network would result in when you speak to them for support. Often, senior leaders themselves are coaches, so you will be able to tap into their expertise and enthusiasm as well.*
- *Be realistic in your vision. You are more likely to get an agreement to hold 20-minute sessions fortnightly than sessions that are long or very frequent.*
- *Hold a launch session to create interest. Collaborative working is key to CoPs, so perhaps invite external partners to participate – for example students' lecturers – they*

might also be interested in setting up coaching training for students within the students'
theory sessions.

- *Identify rooms and times available for people to book coaching sessions; add some*
  training for those who have not coached before. Ensure this includes a few basic
  coaching techniques to allow individuals to quickly coach. You can always add
  training sessions for more sophisticated techniques at a later date.
- *Don't forget to write a basic coaching agreement; allowing all members of your CoP*
  to contribute to the agreement will ensure mutually agreed-upon principles that are
  written and ensure everyone is engaged.
- *Hold regular sessions that can share different techniques for coaching skills and*
  managing the coaching relationships training also discuss areas that went less well, etc.

Equipping students for lifelong learning and self-coaching

It is hoped that a students' positive experience of being coached will underline to them
the importance of lifelong learning. Seeing the fruits of a regular reflective conversation
where the coachee continues to set goals and see transformational change can inspire
individuals to not shy away from future developmental opportunities. The other outcome
is to equip students with reflective tools that they can continue to use beyond the
coaching relationship. This is known as 'self-coaching' – the ability to take a step back
from a situation that requires some consideration and ask the self some important
reflective questions before stepping into action. For example, once a student has had
experience using the TGROW model previously discussed, they might use this model in
the future when faced with a difficult situation with no obvious solutions. Or they may be
encouraged to think again about their strengths when deliberating over a new situation
after the coaching has finished. This is something the coach might want to discuss with
the coachee during their last few coaching sessions when they reflect back over the
coaching experience, but also look to prepare the coachee for learning and development
opportunities beyond the formal coaching experience.

Summary

In this chapter, we have considered:

- What coaching is and how it differs from mentoring, in order to encourage placement
  supervisors to use a coach approach when supporting students in the workplace.
- Where and how a coach approach might be relevant to the placement supervisor role
- Two specific coaching models: TGROW and the Kolb Reflective Cycle
- How coaching might sit within a wider coaching culture in the workplace

References

Aguilar, E (2017) 'Improve youth coaching with one move: Stop talking', *Education Week*, 20 July
2017.
Dwyer, PA, Hunter Revell, SM, Sethares, KA, Ayotte, BJ (2019) 'The influence of psychological
capital, authentic leadership in preceptors, and structural empowerment on new graduate nurse
burnout and turnover intent', *Applied Nursing Research*, 48, pp. 37–44, ISSN 0897-1897

Downey, M (2003) *Effective coaching: Lessons from the coach's coach.* London: Texere.

General Medical Council/Nursing and Midwifery Council (2022) *Candour – openness and honesty when things go wrong.* https://www.gmc-uk.org/ethical-guidance/ethical-guidance-for-doctors/candour---openness-and-honesty-when-things-go-wrong

Grant, L, Kinman, G (2014) 'Emotional resilience in the helping professions and how it can be enhanced', *Health and Social Care Education,* 3(1), pp. 23–34.

Hasson, F, Zhuang-Shuang, LI, Slater, PF, Guo, X-J (2021) 'Resilience, stress and well-being in undergraduate nursing students in China and the UK', *International Journal of Research in Nursing,* 12(1), pp. 11–20, 10.3844/ijrnsp.2021.11.20

HCPC (2017) *Standards of education and training guidance.* London: Health and Care Professions Council.

Ho, HCY, Chan, YC (July 2022) 'The impact of psychological capital on well-being of social workers: A mixed-methods investigation', *Social Work,* 67 (3), pp. 228–238, 10.1093/sw/swac020

Hurley, J, Hutchinson, M, Kozlowski, D, Gadd, M, van Vorst, S (2020) 'Emotional intelligence as a mechanism to build resilience and non-technical skills in undergraduate nurses undertaking clinical placement', *International Journal of Mental Health Nursing,* 29(1), pp. 47–55.

Kolb, DA (1984). *Experiential learning: Experience as the source of learning and development.* Englewood Cliffs, NJ: Prentice Hall.

Linley, P, Harrington, S (2006) 'Playing to your strengths', *The Psychologist,* 19, pp. 86–89

Luthans, F, Avolio, B (2014) 'Brief summary of psychological capital and introduction to the special issue'. *Journal of Leadership & Organizational Studies,* 21 (2).

NMC (2019) *Regulators unite to support reflective practice across health and care.* London: Nursing and Midwifery Council. https://www.nmc.org.uk/news/press-releases/joint-statement-reflective-practice/

NMC (2008) *Standards to support learning and assessment in practice NMC standards for mentors, practice teachers and teachers.* London: Nursing and Midwifery Council.

NMC (2023) *Part 2: Standards for student supervision and assessment.* London: Nursing and Midwifery Council.

NMC/GMC (2022) *Openness and honesty when things go wrong: The professional duty of candour.* London: Nursing & Midwifery Council, General Medical Council. https://www.nmc.org.uk/standards/guidance/the-professional-duty-of-candour/

Perls, F, Hefferline, RF, Goodman, P (1951) *Gestalt therapy: Excitement and growth in the human personality.* New York: Gestalt Journal Press.

Pisanti, R, van der Doef, M, Maes, S, Lombardo, C, Lazzari, D, & Violani, C (2015) 'Occupational coping self-efficacy explains distress and well-being in nurses beyond psychosocial job characteristics', *Frontiers in Psychology,* 6. 10.3389/fpsyg.2015.01143.

Rogers, J (2008) *Coaching skills: A handbook* (2nd ed.). Maidenhead: Open University Press

Seligman, MEP, Csikszentmihalyi, M (2000). 'Positive psychology: An introduction'. *American Psychologist,* 55(1), pp. 5–14, 10.1037/0003-066X.55.1.5

Sun, T, Zhao, XW, Yang, LB, Fan, LH, 2012. 'The impact of psychological capital on job embeddedness and job performance among nurses: a structural equation approach', *Journal of Advanced Nursing,* 68(1), pp. 69–79.

Wenger-Trayner, BE (2015) *Introduction to communities of practice, a brief overview of the concept and its uses.* https://www.wenger-trayner.com/introduction-to-communities-of-practice/

Wenger, E, McDermott, R, Snyder, WM (2002). *Cultivating communities of practice: A guide to managing knowledge.* Boston: Harvard Business School Press Books.

Yusuf, FR, Kumar, A, Goodson-Celerin, W, Lund, T, Davis, J, Kutash, M, Paidas, CN (2018) 'Impact of coaching on the nurse-physician dynamic', *AACN Advanced Critical Care,* 29(3), pp. 259–267.

Chapter 5

Preparing learners for practice-based assessment

Rowena Slope

By the end of this chapter, you will be able to:

1 Explain the difference between formative and summative assessment
2 Discuss the principles of practice-based assessment
3 Understand why there is a failure to fail learners
4 Describe how to undertake a delegated assessment
5 Evaluate the role of patients, clients and service users in assessment

Introduction

In this chapter, we consider how to prepare a range of learners for practice-based assessment. Formative assessments provide students with feedback on how to improve their performance and build confidence for summative assessments where students' knowledge and understanding is formally assessed against a predetermined benchmark. Within nursing and midwifery, quality assurance standards (NMC, 2019) outline the requirements placed on approved education institutions (AEIs) and provide for education standards for Nursing and Midwifery Council (NMC) approved courses, standards for supervision and assessment and standards for individual programmes. The NMC has published standards of proficiency for nurses and midwives as well as standards for competence and essential skills clusters to meet its statutory duties under the Nursing and Midwifery Order (Gov.UK, 2001). If practice assessors are concerned about a learner, they should raise their concern with the student and access support from other educators including academics from the AEI. There may be occasions where it is appropriate for an individual proficiency to be assessed by a practice supervisor instead of a practice assessor, known as a delegated assessment, and this will be discussed later on in the chapter. The NMC Standards for Student Supervision and Assessment (SSSA) (2018) encourage the use of observations from patients and service users to support feedback to learners.

Formative assessment

Formative feedback is defined by Hughes and Quinn (2013, p. 540) as 'assessment that takes place during the learning process in order to modify teaching and learning activities and improve the performance of students'. Oermann *et al.* (2018, p. 171) define formative assessment as judging 'students' progress in developing skills and is focused

DOI: 10.4324/9781003358602-5

on diagnostic feedback without assigning a grade to the evaluation experience. In essence, formative assessments are designed to provide individualised feedback to students regarding their progression without recourse to an assessment benchmark. Formative assessments are not graded and feedback is qualitative in nature, often verbal, face to face and in real time in the clinical practice environment so it has an immediacy and authenticity over summative assessments where feedback may be written, delayed or quantified.

Formative assessments in practice provide opportunities for students to ask questions and seek further clarification and may offer opportunities from others experiencing or witnessing care such as patients or service users, or members of the multi-disciplinary team to provide feedback. Within practice the differentiation between formative and summative assessments are perhaps not as explicitly differentiated as they are in the higher education environment, but they are better integrated and supported by practice portfolios. Practice portfolios allow students to engage in formative assessments in clinical placement with the support of the multi-disciplinary team and aids their critical reflection and developmental learning, allowing them to map their own strengths and limitations.

Students appreciate formative assessments because these can provide them with valuable feedback about how they are progressing and identify any knowledge or skills or behaviours gaps. Arrogante et al. (2021) found that students appreciated formative assessments and that these were effective in improving their performance in summative assessments. Formative assessments allow students more time to relax and think, and to orientate themselves to the conditions under which the summative assessment will take place. They provide valuable individualised feedback on students' strengths and weaknesses, and how to improve their performance in the summative assessment. The greatest benefits of formative assessments are perhaps as a diagnostic tool for student and assessor to support future learning and assessment.

Summative assessment

Summative assessments are used to evaluate what a student has learned and comes at the end of instruction (Oermann et al., 2018, p. 171). In the university setting, summative assignments are often associated with essays and examinations but summative assessments can involve assessment of skill and proficiencies in the clinical practice setting. The assessment is set out beforehand and the goals made explicit to the learner before they undertake the skill. The students are aware that they are being assessed and they must proceed without comment and feedback is often quantified and graded either pass or fail. This transparency is important for trust between the learner and the assessor. Formative assessments are often designed to prepare students for their summative assessment and the practice portfolio is designed in this way. Summative assessments may be undertaken by a single assessor, but in an accredited nursing programme there will be oversight by academic assessors and higher education institutional arrangements. The assessor should ensure that they have a good understanding of the assessment process, the skill to be assessed, and to ensure that grade and feedback are documented and provided to the student in a timely fashion. Summative assessments must be objective, fair and evidence based. There should be consistency between the learning outcomes, assignment task, marking criteria, grade and feedback.

Summative assessments are useful because they offer a standard of achievement that the learner can aim for. Assessment of nursing and midwifery students, for example, plays an important role in maintaining consistent standards of the profession and ensuring that newly qualified nurses and midwives are proficient in their clinical skills. Summative assessments can provide an indication of what has been learned and constructive feedback and grading can provide students with vital information of whether they have met the required standard. Oversight is required to ensure that summative feedback is fair and can give an indication of the quality of the teaching itself. Feedback may be immediate and verbal but should always be formalised and accurately documented. Students should be given time to consider their feedback and the opportunity to seek further clarification of anything that is unclear.

NMC standards and assessment

The NMC (2023) Part 1: Standards Framework for Nursing, Part 2: Standards for Student Supervision and Assessment, and Part 3: Standards for pre-registration for nursing programmes make reference to the importance of continuous feedback; the opportunities for student self-reflection; and the importance of ensuring that diversity and equality legislation is honoured. The NMC (2023, p. 49) has made it clear that assessment in practice should be undertaken by direct observation as well as evidence gathered from indirect observation such as via practice supervisors. However even summative assessments can be simulated if the practice experience is not available (2023, p. 49). Essentially, Practice Assessment Documents such as the MYEPAD, Pan London PAD or OPAL are formative in nature until the point of the final assessment, assessment of proficiencies and the OAR. The NMC principles of practice-based assessment do not quantify how many times a student can be formatively assessed but focus instead on ensuring fairness, partnership, reflection and safety. However, these should be sufficiently informative and transparent so that students have a good idea of how they will perform in the final summative assessment for their clinical placement, and know where and how to get further support should they need it, such as from practice educators.

Practice-based assessments are often a 'public endeavour' and may take place in the presence of other qualified healthcare professionals, support workers and administrators, patients and service users, members of the public including visiting family and religious personnel (Quinn & Peters, 2017, p. 358). Practice assessors should be aware the presence of this audience can hinder or enhance performance (Hughes and Quinn, 2016, p. 358). Nevertheless, the practice environment by its very nature lends authenticity to the assessment, whether summative or formative, and provides the context within which the student will be expected to perform independently once qualified.

Activity 1

Consider your experience of working within and supervising learners in your current role:

- What kind of formative assessments might be useful to support learners with their summative assessment in your practice environment?
- What type of feedback from formative assessments would learners find helpful in identifying how to improve their practice performance?

- How would you support a student who was anxious about being assessed in a public place?
- Which practice assessments would lend themselves to simulation?

Principles of practice-based assessments

AEIs work in partnership with practice placement and practice learning providers to deliver educational programmes approved by the professional standard regulatory bodies, such as the Nursing and Midwifery Council (NMC). AEIs must meet the requirements of the NMC Quality Assurance framework (2019) in order to be approved as an AEI. This process ensures that nurses, midwives and nursing associates receive appropriate education and training that meets NMC standards, thus ensuring the protection of the public and ongoing support of students.

The Standards Framework for Nursing and Midwifery Education was updated in January 2023 and supplemented by additional safeguarding provisions. Since the removal of the European Union (EU) Directive 2005/36/EC, prospective nursing or midwifery students no longer need to demonstrate that they have 10–12 years of general education. This means that young people under the age of 18 may in some circumstances be eligible to join an NMC-approved programme. The safeguarding measures are designed to protect students under the age of 18 by ensuring that they have sufficient maturity to participate in the course, that consideration is given to their age when arranging shift patterns, and that individualised student journeys are created to meet their needs (NMC, 2023).

Standards are designed to be flexible and creative to allow for the delivery of education and training to nursing, midwifery and nursing associate students across different institutions and care settings. The NMC (2023) standards are set out in three parts: Part 1: Standards Framework for Nursing and Midwifery Education; Part 2: Standards for Student Supervision and Assessment and Part 3: Programme Standards. The latter provides for standards for pre-registration nursing, pre-registration midwifery, pre-registration nursing associates, prescribing, post-registration and return to practice. The standards contain the principles for practice-based assessments.

Part 1 of the Standards Framework for Nursing and Midwifery is organised around five headings: learning culture, educational governance and quality, student empowerment, education and assessors and curricula and assessment. A summary of these follows.

Learning culture

These standards state that learning must prioritise safety, and that education and training must be valued in the respective learning environment. The NMC standards (2019) make it clear that all assessments including formative should be 'fair, impartial, transparent, fosters good relations between individuals and diverse groups, and is compliant with equalities and human rights legislation' (2018, 1.10, p. 6).

Practice-based assessors are responsible for ensuring that practice-based assessments are evidence-based, objective and fair and incorporate different learning styles, cultural backgrounds and communication styles as well as being mindful of students' previous level of achievement. Practice assessment should be continuous, and students provided with timely feedback. Learning environments should meet the needs of a service users, students, and other stakeholders working collaboratively together. They must provide a learning context where students can meet the outcomes and proficiencies of their respective courses as well as meet the NMC's Standards for Student Supervision and Assessment contained in Part 2.

Educational governance and quality

These standards are designed to ensure that education providers comply with current regulation and legislation and must consider the diverse needs of students and stakeholders and be designed in partnership (2018, 2.2, p. 7). This partnership approach ensures that providers share the responsibility for practice and theory supervision, learning and assessment (2018, 2.5, p. 7).

These standards also cover recruitment, recognition of prior learning, regulatory compliance, the quality of external examiners, the safety of the learning environment and have the potential to identify any areas for improvement.

Student empowerment

These standards ensure that students have access to varied learning opportunities and resources to enable them to meet the proficiencies and professional behaviours of their respective programme. A commitment to lifelong and reflective learning is embedded in these standards. It further provides for the provision of timely and accurate information on placement and university teaching, use of technology including simulated learning environments, and appropriate supervision. This includes a nominated practice assessor in placement and a nominated academic assessor in the AEI, protected learning time in placement, pastoral support and constructive feedback.

Education and assessors

This standard mandates that everyone involved in providing education and training to students should be suitably qualified, prepared and skilled. They should collaborate with other colleagues and partner organisations to deliver supervision and assessment. It was reported that some students who experienced the transition between the old and new standards mourned the loss of the mentor, although this may also have been due to difficulties associated with managing transitions, while the benefits of the new standards included drawing upon a wider team of support (Highe, 2020).

Curricula and assessment

It is the responsibility of the NMC to establish the appropriate curricula and assessments to ensure that students can practice safely in their chosen field. The curricular are designed to meet the proficiency and programme outcomes and should be consistent with the health and social care agenda. Students should be assessed across their practice settings and assessment mapped to the curricular while practice and theory components should be weighted across the programme without compensation mechanisms if students are deficient in one area.

Activity 2

Read through Part 1 of the Standards Framework for Nursing and Midwifery (NMC, 2023) or the professional standard regulatory body guidance relevant to your role as an assessor. Consider your current practice learning environment:

- How does this learning environment ensure the safety of learners, patients, service users, family members, clinical staff and other stakeholders?
- What are the key legislative requirements relevant to your practice learning environment?
- What kind of varied learning experiences are available in your practice learning environment?
- How would you support a young person aged 17?

Proficiencies and competencies

Article 5(2) of the Nursing and Midwifery Order (2001) required the NMC to draw up standards of proficiency for admittance onto the register for all fields of nursing and midwives. In response, the NMC published *The Future Nurse: Standards of Proficiency for Registered Nurses* (2018) and *Standards of Proficiency for Midwives* (2019). The standards must be regularly updated to respond to changing demographics, public health, technology and developments in the evidence base and are designed to produce autonomous professionals who can work in collaboration with the multidisciplinary team. The proficiencies for nurses are structured around seven platforms: being an accountable professional; promoting health and preventing ill health; assessing needs and planning care; providing and evaluating care; leading and managing care and working in teams; improving safety and quality of care and coordinating care. These platforms are enhanced by a further two annexes on communication and relationship management skills, and nursing procedures.

The proficiencies for midwives have a global outlook and are based around six domains: being an accountable, autonomous, professional midwife; safe and effective midwifery care; promoting and providing continuity of care and carer; universal care for all women and new-born infants; additional care for women and newborn infants with complications; promoting excellence, the midwife as colleague, scholar and leader and the midwife as a skilled practitioner (NMC, 2019).

The reception upon release of these proficiencies was generally positive. Meegan *et al.* (2020) welcomed the commitment to improve childhood health in line with UNICEF's Baby Friendly Initiative. However, Warrender (2022) raised concerns that the nurse proficiency standards did not reflect what mental health student nurses needed to know.

There are four general competencies that apply to all fields of nursing (child, adult, mental health and learning disability) that have remained the same since they were published in 2010. These include professional values; communication and interpersonal skills; nursing practice and decision making and leadership, management and team-working. These competencies incorporate general knowledge and understanding as well as field-specific competencies that nurses must demonstrate before they can apply to join the register. These competencies ensure that nurses can deliver high quality care, uphold the professional expectations embedded within the NMC (2023) and protect the public.

The publication of the competencies was undertaken to improve professional transparency following the publication of *More Care, Less Pathway: A Review of the Liverpool Care Pathway* (Independent Review of the Liverpool Care Pathway, 2013). These competencies are supported by five essential skills clusters and feed into the nursing degree programme: care, compassion and communication; organisational aspects of care; infection, prevention and control; nutrition and fluid management and medicines management (NMC, 2023, p. 20).

Similarly, there are Standards for Competence for Registered Midwives that must be adhered to throughout the registrant's career and these, too, remain unchanged since 2009. The Standards for Competence are effective midwifery practice; professional and ethical practice; developing the individual midwife and others and achieving quality care through evaluation and research. The essential skills clusters are communication; initial consultation between the woman and the midwife; normal labour and birth; initiation and continuance of breastfeeding and medicines management (NMC, 2019, p. 13).

Activity 3

Reflect on the proficiencies in your area of practice and consider:

- How are changing demographics impacting your patients or service users?
- What technological advancements have been introduced and how you will use these to support learners?
- What practice experiences support the development of autonomous practitioners?
- How has the evidence base changed and informed your area of practice in the last three years?

Failure to fail

Failure to fail refers to the passing of learners in clinical practice who have not met the appropriate professional standards according to their stage of development. This phenomenon is recognised across different healthcare professions, not just in nursing and midwifery, and is a feature regardless of the clinical practice educational model in place (Hughes *et al.*, 2019). Failure to fail has international significance in an increasingly globalised work where many healthcare professionals migrate to work in countries different from the one they trained in. The passing of learners who have not met the required knowledge, professional behaviours and clinical proficiencies goes beyond the traditional failure to fail dilemma whereby a teacher is conflicted about failing a student because it may reflect poorly upon them. This is because in nursing, health and social care, incompetent practitioners pose a risk to the public and can bring their profession into disrepute. It is also detrimental to the learner and future professional who are more likely to be involved in a negative incident in practice. To address this problem, different models of supervision have been tried across different countries, including the use of individual mentors, cohorts, wider peer groups, and stakeholder engagement (Hughes *et al.*, 2019).

Instances of failure to fail are known to occur across different countries and there is growing evidence based on this subject matter in the United Kingdom and beyond (Hunt, 2019; Hunt *et al.*, 2016). This has been a problem reported before the introduction of the new NMC standards, which were designed to address some of these concerns. For example, the introduction of practice assessors was designed in part to alleviate the pressures on mentors who may have found it difficult to fail a learner they had built up a relationship with. Meanwhile, Academic Assessors would be able to take a more objective overview that incorporated academic and clinical practice elements, and therefore make a more informed judgement regarding learner performance. Assessment tools and criteria are important strategies for effective assessment of learners, according to a systematic review conducted by Immonen et al. (2019), as well as individualised feedback and reflection that together increase the reliability and objectivity of the assessment process. The new standards aimed to incorporate these elements.

One of the tensions that has emerged from the commercialisation of higher education is that most learners pay university fees and increasingly high costs of living in order to study. Learners on healthcare registrant courses have limited opportunity to undertake paid work compared to traditional higher education students. AEIs are under pressure to increase student numbers to secure income with the inevitable consequences that weaker students are being admitted into nursing courses. This has increased the potential for students to experience 'practical, psychological and emotional hurdles' (Cassidy et al., 2020).

A survey conducted by Hughes et al. (2019) discovered that almost a quarter of the clinical nurse educators they had questioned had 'given the benefit of the doubt' to students they had concerns about. There were reports of intimidation as a factor from a small cohort of student nurses although this appeared to be a less significant problem. However, a total of 44% of participants felt that they did not have sufficient time to adequately assess students (Hughes et al., 2019).

Programmes such as nursing or midwifery represent a blend of science and art and the complexity of assessing these learners has been of concern for many years (Immonen et al., 2019). Hunt (2012) found that the ratio of failure in theory compared to practice was significantly different, although this was undertaken under previous nurse education standards. Cassidy et al. (2020) emphasise the value of supportive arrangements with the local AEI in the case of practice assessors having particular concern about a learner. The use of an action plan is often perceived as punitive by students and practice assessors, but they can be a vital tool in ensuring transparency of feedback and clarity regarding supportive action required from clinical placement and the AEI. They can help direct the learner to appropriate actions that will improve their performance, such as engagement with a practice educator.

The NMC (2023) makes it clear that practice assessors have a responsibility to raise concerns regarding any students' competence and/or conduct and that this should be undertaken in a 'timely and responsible' way. Although it does not clarify what timely or responsible means. The NMC (2023) also makes it clear that is the responsibility of the AEI to have protocols in place to support practice supervisors.

Activity 4

Reflect on a recent learner who appeared to have encountered barriers to meeting their expected level of knowledge and understanding:

- What support would you want from the AEI?

- At what point would you initiate an action plan?
- What resources did you signpost the learner to?
- What questions would you ask a learner to illicit any barriers to learning?

Undertaking a delegated assessment

There are occasions when an individual proficiency may be assessed by a practice supervisor rather than a practice assessor and this is permitted by the NMC Standards for Student Supervision and Assessment (2023).

Under the section 'What is current knowledge and experience':

If a registered professional is competent in an area of practice, they should be able to supervise and support a nursing or midwifery student for that area, providing feedback on their progress towards, and achievement of, proficiencies and skills. The practice supervisor's knowledge and experience should enable the student to meet their learning needs and outcomes and enhance the student learning experiences.

Furthermore, in the section 'What do practice supervisors do?' the guidance states that practice supervisors should be 'providing direct feedback to nursing and midwifery students on their conduct and achievement of proficiencies and skills, including where they don't think the achievement has been met, or could be improved on' and a 'key part of giving feedback is adding relevant observations on the student's conduct, proficiency and achievement to the student's record(s) of achievement' (NMC, 2023).

Additional clarification is outlined in the section on practice supervisors contributing to recommendations for progression. The guidance states:

'Contributing to student assessments can take different forms depending on the role of the practice supervisor in student learning, the stage of learning, student competence, and other considerations. It can include: direct communication with practice and academic assessors to share their views on student achievement, underachievement or areas to continue to work on; inputting into student documentation with their views on student achievement' (NMC, 2023).

There may be situations where the practice supervisor has more qualifications and experience to assess a particular proficiency than the practice assessor, so it may make sense to have this proficiency delegated to the supervisor. Practice assessors are expected to review diverse evidence from the wider multi-professional team as well as the practice supervisor, patients, service users and the public when they assess students. The SSSA (2023) is designed to be flexible, innovative and outcome focused and suitable for use across all platforms and settings, and delegating assessments to suitably qualified practice supervisors, assuming that standards are maintained is within the spirit of this.

Therefore, the practice supervisor can record the achievement of individual proficiencies in the assessment document, but it remains the responsibility of the practice assessor to be sure that the level of achievement is maintained at the point of assessment. The practice assessor is making the overall assessment decision, and retains the right to overrule the supervisor's record of achievement in the assessment document for the individual proficiencies if they are concerned that it has not met this standard.

Roles of patients, clients and service users

The NMC (SSSA, 2023) allows for and encourages observations from 'anyone who has taken part in the student's education' and this includes patients, clients and service users. The new standards also envisaged feedback from service users in the assessment process. During the approval process for AEI to train nurses, nursing associates and midwives, AEIs are required to demonstrate how they incorporate patient and service user experience into their courses. Many AEIs use service users to help review courses and interview prospective students. Feedback from those receiving care can inform feedback to students on their conduct and competence.

Indeed, practice assessment documents include pages designed for patients, clients and service users to provide feedback and provide space for written comments, numerical scales and space for drawings. Observations from patients, clients and service users can provide a unique form of feedback that provides an authenticity and realism to feedback that can be helpful to the student. However, patients, clients and service users have the right not to be cared for or observed by a student and consent should be requested before care or observation takes place (NMC, 2018a). This may not always be possible in environments where patients are unconscious, such as a Resuscitation Department or Intensive Care Unit, or where patients have reduced capacity, but sensitivity and tact are still important.

It may be advisable for the practice supervisor or assessor to seek feedback on student performance without the presence of the student, to ensure that feedback is honest and consent gained for feedback to be documented. Students may ask service users to document directly in their Practice Assessment Documents, but some AEIs have produced their own leaflet. The University of the West of England has produced a leaflet entitled 'Patient/Carer Feedback: enhancing learning for student nurses'. This leaflet seeks both quantitative and qualitative feedback and asks patients/carers to evaluate student nurses on five criteria and can be found in the reference list.

Activity 5

Design a leaflet or form that can be used in your practice area that incorporates the five criteria from the University of the West of England's patient/carer feedback leaflet:

1   How would you rate the nursing care provided by the student?
2   How compassionate was the student's care?
3   How respectfully did the student treat you?
4   How well did the student listen to you?
5   How clearly did the student communicate with you?

Summary

This chapter has provided an overview of arrangements for preparing a range of students, learners and apprentices for practice-based assessments. It has explained the difference between formative and summative assessment, and the different ways these support the learner. It has discussed the principles of practice-based assessment, including partnership arrangements with AEIs. Key proficiencies and competencies ensure that registrants are suitably qualified to deliver care quality and safeguard the public. Finally, this chapter outlined reasons for failure to fail, and how feedback from patients and service users can be used to support learners in practice.

References

Arrogante, O, González-Romero, GM, López-Torre, EM, et al. (2021) 'Comparing formative and summative simulation-based assessment in undergraduate nursing students: Nursing competency acquisition and clinical simulation satisfaction', BMC Nursing, 20, p. 92, 10.1186/s12912-021-00614-2

Cassidy, S, Coffey, M, Murphy, F (2020) 'Transparency of assessment decision-making when students are not meeting required levels of proficiency in clinical practice', Nurse Education in Practice, 43, 10.1016/j.nepr.2020.102711

GOV.UK (2001) Nursing & Midwifery 2001. https://www.legislation.gov.uk/uksi/2002/253/contents/made

Highe, L (2020) 'The cultural change from mentor to practice assessor/supervisor', Evidence-Based Nursing. https://blogs.bmj.com/ebn/2020/02/16/the-cultural-change-from-mentor-to-practice-assessor-supervisor/ (Accessed: 23 May 2023).

Hughes, LJ, Mitchell, M, Johnston, AN (2016) 'Failure to fail' in nursing – A catch phrase or a real issue? A systematic integrative literature review', Nurse Education in Practice, 20, pp. 54–63, 10.1016/j.nepr.2016.06.009. Epub 29 Jun 2016. PMID: 27428804.

Hunt, LA (2019) 'Developing a 'core of steel': The key attributes of effective practice assessors', British Journal of Nursing, 28(22), pp. 1478–1484.

Hunt, LA, McGee, P, Gutteridge, R, Hughes, M (2012) 'Assessment of student nurses in practice: A comparison of theoretical and practical assessment results in England', Nurse Education Today, 32(4), pp. 351–355.

Hunt, LA, McGee, P, Gutteridge, R, Hughes, M. (2016) 'Failing securely: The processes and support which underpin English nurse mentors' assessment decisions regarding under-performing students', Nurse Education Today, 39, pp. 79–86, 10.1016/j.nedt.2016.01.011. Epub 28 Jan 2016. PMID: 27006036.

Hughes, LJ, Mitchell, ML, Johnston, ANB. (2019) 'Just how bad does it have to be? Industry and academic assessors' experiences of failing to fail – A descriptive study', Nurse Education Today, 76, pp. 206–215, 10.1016/j.nedt.2019.02.011

Immonen, K, Oikarainen, A, Tomietto, M, Kääriäinen, M, Tuomikoski, A-N, Kaučič, BM, Filej, B, Riklikiene, O, Vizcaya-Moreno, MF, Perez-Cañaveras, RM, Raeve, P de, Mikkonen, K (2019) 'Assessment of nursing students' competence in clinical practice: A systematic review of reviews', International Journal of Nursing Studies, 100, 10.1016/j.ijnurstu.2019.103414

Independent Review of the Liverpool Care Pathway (2013) More care, less pathway: A review of the liverpool care pathway. https://assets.publishing.service.gov.uk/government/uploads/system/uploads/attachment (Accessed: 23 May 2023).

NMC (2018a) Future nurse: Standards of proficiency for registered nurses. https://www.nmc.org.uk/globalassets/sitedocuments/education-standards/future-nurs e-proficiencies.pdf (Accessed: 22 May 2023).

NMC (2018b) Realising professionalism: Standards for education and training. Part 1: Standards framework for nursing and midwifery education. https://www.nmc.org.uk//globalassets/sitedocuments/standards-of-proficiency/standards-framework-for-nursing-and-midwifery-education/education-framework.pdf (Accessed: 23 May 2023).

NMC (2018c) Standards for competence for midwives. https://www.nmc.org.uk/globalassets/sitedocuments/standards/nmc-standards-for-competence-for-registered-midwives.pdf (Accessed: 23 May 2023).

NMC (2018d) Standards for competence for registered nurses. https://www.nmc.org.uk/globalassets/sitedocuments/standards/nmc-standards-for-competence-for-registered-nurses.pdf (Accessed: 23 May 2023).

NMC (2018e) Standards of proficiency for midwives. https://www.nmc.org.uk//globalassets/sitedocuments/standards/standards-of-proficiency-for-midwives.pdf (Accessed: 23 May 2023).

NMC (2019) Quality assurance framework for nursing, midwifery and nursing associate education, London, Nursing & Midwifery Council. https://www.nmc.org.uk/education/quality-assurance-of-education/how-we-quality-assure/#:~:text=Quality%20assurance%20(QA)%20is%20the,programmes%20and%20monitoring%20those%20programmes.

NMC (2019) Standards of proficiency for midwives, London, Nursing & Midwifery Council. https://www.nmc.org.uk/standards/standards-for-midwives/standards-of-proficiency-for-midwives/

Meegan, S (2020) 'Revised standards of proficiencies for midwives: An opportunity to influence childhood health?' *British Journal of Midwifery*. https://www.britishjournalofmidwifery.com//content/clinical-practice/revised-standards-of-proficiencies-for-midwives-an-opportunity-to-influence-childhood-health/ (Accessed: 23 May 2023).

NMC (2023) *Safeguarding Students*. Available at: https://www.nmc.org.uk/standards/guidance/supporting-information-for-our-education-and-training-standards/safeguarding-students/ (Accessed: 23 May 2023).

NMC (2023) *Standards for education and training. Part 2: Standards for student supervision and assessment*. https://www.nmc.org.uk/standards-for-education-and-training/standards-for-student-supervision-and-assessment/ (Accessed: 22 May 2023).

NMC (2023) Standards framework for nursing and midwifery education Part 1 of our standards for education and training, London, Nursing & Midwifery Council. https://www.nmc.org.uk/standards-for-education-and-training/standards-framework-for-nursing-and-midwifery-education/

NMC (2023) Standards for pre-registration nursing programmes, London, Nursing & Midwifery Council. https://www.nmc.org.uk/standards/standards-for-nurses/standards-for-pre-registration-nursing-programmes/

NMC (2023) Standards for student supervision and assessment, London, Nursing & Midwifery Council. https://www.nmc.org.uk/standards-for-education-and-training/standards-for-student-supervision-and-assessment/

Oermann MH, De Gagne JC, Phillips BC (eds) (2018) *Teaching in nursing and role of the educator: The complete guide to best practice in teaching, evaluation, and curriculum development (2nd ed.).* New York, NY: Springer Publishing Company, LLC.

Quinn, BL, Peters, A (2017) 'Strategies to reduce nursing student test anxiety: A literature review', *Journal of Nursing Education*, 56(3), pp. 145–151.

Warrender, D (2022) 'NMC proficiency standards are an assault on mental health nursing', *Mental Health Practice*. https://rcni.com/mental-health-practice/opinion/comment/nmc-proficiency-standards-are-assault-on-mental-health-nursing-189961 (Accessed: 22 May 2023).

Chapter 6

Learning conversations

Mark Wareing

By the end of this chapter, you will be able to:

1 Identify when learning is transformational.
2 Describe at least three strategies to support peer-to-peer learning.
3 Explain the key characteristics of effective feedback.
4 Analyse the value of conversations that matter.
5 Explore the role of emotion arising from learning conversations.

Introduction

The quality of practice and workplace learning is contingent on effective communication between all workers, particularly if learning and working are to be coincident within rich and rewarding learning environments. In this chapter, we will explore how practice supervisors, educators and assessors can facilitate learning using reflective, developmental 'conversations that matter' to ensure that learning is a transformational experience. This is intended to move away from a purely transactional approach, where supervisors and assessors merely engage with learners for the purpose of delivering feedback; either verbally or in written form. Additionally, we will identify the role of peer-assisted learning and protected learning opportunities to enable students, apprentices and trainees to develop their knowledge, understanding and skills in support of learning for all. There are a large number of activities within this chapter that have a particular focus on the importance of effective written as well as verbal feedback, although you are not expected to complete them all!

Transformational learning

Students, apprentices and learners commencing training, programmes of study and apprenticeships are often encountering some of the most vivid developmental learning experiences of their lives, where threshold knowledge and experiences shape their identity and the professional that they decide to become. The trajectory of learning starts with the trainee being given an ascribed identity as a nursing, midwifery, social work or therapies student, leading eventually to an achieved identity at graduation signified by their entry to a profession and registration with a regulatory body. To what extent can practice supervisors, assessors and educators make sense of the depth and richness of practice learning experiences and understand their impact on the student, learner or apprentice?

DOI: 10.4324/9781003358602-6

One theoretical framework that is particularly sensitive to vivid and meaningful experiences is the concept of transformational learning. Illeris (2014) describes six key principles that characterise learning experiences that are said to be personally transformational for learners within a range of settings. A truly transformational learning experience must be purposeful and include learning processes that are heuristic, whereby learning is facilitated through discovery. The facilitator needs to ensure that the learning experience or environment is sufficiently safe for the learner to be given the opportunity to confront power and engage with difference, which in turn requires the student, trainee or apprentice to use their imagination to the point where they are 'led to the edge'. Being led to the edge may require the facilitator to identify the current limits of their learner's understanding, knowledge and skills and to have their values challenged. Transformational learning experiences need to foster reflection and include opportunities for learners to observe effective practitioners and model their behaviours.

In summary, the characteristics of transformational learning are:

1   Experiences that are purposeful, including heuristic processes that enable learning through discovery.
2   Opportunities for learners to confront power and engage in and with difference.
3   Learning that utilises imaginative processes.
4   When learners have been 'led to the edge'.
5   Experiences that foster reflection.
6   Time for the observation of effective people and to model behaviours.

(Illeris, 2014, pp. 10–11)

Activity 1

Think about the clinical, therapeutic or practice area where you work and the services and interventions that it provides:

1   What opportunities are there for learning by discovery?
2   How comfortable would you be if a learner highlighted issues of power and difference that they felt related to the patient, client and service user experience?
3   How might learners be 'led to the edge' in such a way that patient and client safety is not compromised?
4   What particular experiences appear to foster reflection amongst learners and why might this be so?
5   How comfortable are you at modelling behaviours before students, apprentices and trainees? What might they see, find useful, or less useful?

The role of the practice supervisor, assessor and educator is to not only facilitate high-quality supportive and safe learning experiences, but to identify evidence of what is transformed within the learner. Illeris (2014, pp. 25–27) suggests that the learner may demonstrate change when the learning experience has had a psychotherapeutic effect, which may have occurred through a particularly deep and emotive experience, perhaps when practice learning has re-framed an earlier significant event connected with practice. In such a situation, the practice supervisor, assessor or educator needs to exercise considerable care and sensitivity, as the learner may need debriefing or signposting to support services outside of the immediate practice area, placement or organisation. If the student has a pre-existing or an enduring mental health condition, an assessment of the extent to which the learner might be seeking a therapeutic benefit from the clinical area may need to be considered alongside the decision to change the placement. Ordinary cognitive changes may be evident within the learner, particularly if they have developed a deeper appreciation of decision-making and the role of intuitive judgement within client- and patient-facing interaction and assessment. A transformational learning experience may be particularly empowering if a learner's consciousness has been raised and enabled their understanding of power, situatedness, politics or positionality. Change may also be seen within learners' cognitive structures, in relation to their ability to make sense of the immediate practice environment, their intentionality and response to and engagement with artefacts, objects and equipment. This particular dimension of transformational learning may present a particular challenge to the learner with a special learning difference such as dyspraxia, particularly when they are being required to master technical skills alongside procedural knowledge and develop spatial awareness. Similarly, students with a special learning need associated with autism or learners with a social anxiety disorder may need particular support strategies to enable them to learn through interaction, sufficient for transformational changes in the self, identity and the biography of the learner to be realised. Chapters 7 and 15 focus on student/apprentice health and wellbeing and how to support students with special learning differences, respectively. Finally, evidence that transformational learning has occurred is when a student, trainee or apprentice is able to recontextualise their learning through a discussion of the development of society as their underlying frame of reference. This process is particularly relevant when learners are engaging with global and public health perspectives, including the local health economy, sustainability, injustice or health policy.

Activity 2

Using Illeris's evidence for transformational learning, as described in the last section, identifies a vivid personal learning experience that may have had a psychotherapeutic, cognitive effect or changed your understanding of power and the nature of society.

Holding conversations that matter

In the last section, we explored the dimensions of transformational learning and how practice supervisors, assessors and educators can analyse the outcomes of facilitated learning experiences. It is evident that communication and communicative action is at the centre of all participatory and opportunistic learning experiences and activities. Our attention will now focus upon the quality of developmental reflective discussion, or more simply, the activity of holding a 'conversation that matters'. Traditionally, within coaching, where the learner is supported in their journey from one destination to another; and mentoring, where the mentee's thinking is the primary focus, the quality of the relationship between the coach, mentor and learner is fundamental to the meeting of learning outcomes. Within such relationships, students, trainees and apprentices are encouraged to learn from the experience of existing and novel situations, drawing on, interpreting and integrating the information these present in order to support the development of new behaviours (Foster-Turner, 2006, pp. 3–4). This recommendation highlights that whilst the inclination of the learner is to focus on new areas, there is much that can and should be learnt from seemingly similar or regular client interactions and episodes of care. Similarly, for the practice supervisor, assessor and educator, their engagement with students, apprentices and learners creates an opportunity to take a fresh look at every day procedures, practices and interactions. Raelin (2008, pp. 172–173) comments that 'what makes each relationship unique as a work-based learning approach, is the interest of the parties in mutual reflection and learning … there is much for the coach to learn as the participant'. Therefore, it is important for practice supervisors, educators and assessors to be able to facilitate productive reflection to ensure that learners can reflect on their learning and receive feedback from their supervisor and ensure that personal learning objectives have been met. This requires a collaborative approach within a relationship characterised by mutual reflection, development and learning. The use of a learning log sheet (see Box 1) can enable students to identify learning objectives at the start of each working day, shift or other period of supervised practice and gather evidence to discuss with their practice supervisor or assessor that can link with their practice assessment documentation.

Box I   Learning log sheet

You will recall that in Chapter 4 we looked at the principles of coaching, which requires practice supervisors and educators to encourage learners to set their own goals, with the coach providing a 'steer' where learning objectives are negotiated by the student, not imposed on the student. If conversations are to occur that truly matter, the practice supervisor and educator need to be non-judgemental and allow the learner to come to their own judgement about their performance, interactions and clinical care. This can be facilitated by encouraging the learner to make a judgement on the basis of evidence or, in the absence of research, to determine the best practice.

Using a questioning approach

Adopting a coaching technique will enable the practice supervisor and educator to facilitate thinking using open questioning; where questions start with verbs such as *where, what, how* and *why* that lead to discussion, rather than 'closed' questions that require a yes or no answer. Using framing and re-framing conversationally is a particularly useful coaching device (Claridge and Lewis, 2005). Framing questions tend to be short and can be deployed to enable learning to occur whilst in the flow of work or to enable reflection-in-action (Schön, 1991). For example, practice supervisors and educators can ask their learners:

1 *What might be the outcome* [for the client, carer, relative, service user]?
2 *What do you want* [from this episode of care, learning experience]?
3 *What really matters to you, in all of this* [interaction, meeting, episode, visit]?

Useful framing questions can also be facilitated when the supervisor or educator paraphrases that which the learner has shared and conveys active listening:

1   *So, what you are saying is … ?*
2   *Can we retrace out steps?*
3   *Okay, but how would it be if … ?*

Reframing questions tend to be longer and designed to be retrospective to promote reflecting-on-action (Schön, 1991) and are perhaps better used during periods of reflection at the end of a particular learning experience, shift or the working day and include:

1   *Now that we have reflected on this incident together, I wonder if we can look at this from another angle/in somebody else's shoes by imagining that …*
2   *On the one hand, I hear you saying this … but on the other hand I hear you also saying something else …*
3   *If you had three wishes …*
4   *If this were a story, what is the part that needs to be told next?*
5   *Okay, so what happens next?*

Reframing questions can be enlivened through the use of metaphors that may convey an illustrative device or visual image to deepen the learners' reflective thinking ahead of their response, whilst giving the questioner time to re-group and subsequent contribution to the discussion:

1   I can see that you are surprised/puzzled. Tell me, what is the *muddiest* point?
2   You appear to have had a vivid learning experience today. Tell me, what will you *take away* from the experience?

Peer-to-peer learning

In order for practice learning to be enhanced and enriched, models of peer-assisted learning have been developed within clinical and therapeutic environments that expand placement capacity by providing a supportive framework that increases the number of learners within a practice area. The coaching and peer-assisted learning (C-PAL) model is one example of how groups of students are able to adopt a team approach to their learning that enables senior students to gain valuable clinical management and leadership experience and enhance student satisfaction (Wareing et al., 2018). Table 6.1 provides an outline of five models that facilitate coaching and peer-assisted learning and can be used in a range of clinical and therapeutic areas. Students can be supported by a coach whilst looking after a group of patients, clients or service users, or be placed in pairs (dyads) or groups of threes (triads) or fours (quads). The primary goal of each model of peer-assisted learning is to ensure student's practice learning and working becomes coincident. This requires support and timely intervention from a coach who coaches with their 'hands behind their back', intervening when necessary to maintain patient safety and sustain peer-learning. Learner triads or quads can be established where senior or final year students lead junior students in developmental reflective conversations around

Table 6.1 Models that facilitate coaching and peer-assisted learning

Models	Description
Classic C-PAL	A **mix** of **first-, second- or third-year students** look after **a 'bay' or group of patients or clients** within an **in-patient setting**. Final-year students may coordinate care, under supervision, and with input from a **coach** who supports all learners with 'their hands behind their back' only intervening when necessary to maintain patient safety and ensuring that there are regular **'huddling'** meetings where students come together to share and explain their care intentions.
Horizontal C-PAL	A **group** comprising of **students** from the **same year** or **cohort** look after **a 'bay' or group of patients or clients** within an **in-patient setting**. Students are supervised by a **coach** who supports all learners and intervenes to support, direct, question and maintain patient safety. The coach initiates regular **'huddling'**.
Learner Dyad	A **pair of students**, either within the **same ward, department or clinical/therapeutic team** <u>or</u> located in **two different care settings**, meet either **daily, several times a week or weekly** to engage in **productive reflection**, set new learning objectives review **daily learning log sheets**. Learner dyads might be created where students in different placements prepare each other to 'swap over'.
Learner Triad	**Three students**, either within the **same ward, department or clinical/therapeutic team** or located in **different care settings** meet **weekly** to engage in **productive reflection**, set new learning objectives review **daily learning log sheets**. Students may be a **mixture of first, second or third years**. Where a **final-year student** is present, their role would normally be to **provide peer coaching** to junior students and **lead the reflective discussions**.

a particular topic, area of practice, case study or episode of care. Additionally, learner dyads can also facilitate peer learning between students whose placement areas are in different locations and are particularly useful for students undertaking rotational placements, where students can prepare each other ahead of the rotation.

The implementation of a peer-assisted learning model requires preparation to ensure that all members of staff and service users understand the rationale for the peer-to-peer learning; not least as some models are contingent on an increase in students, which some patients or clients may find challenging. Most clinical or therapeutic practice areas will have an education link or nominated person responsible for students, who should have responsibility for and access to the placement's educational audit. This document normally contains information on the placement capacity, which will enable initial planning to commence and inform decision-making regarding the selection of an appropriate model of peer learning. Additionally, practice staff will need to consider how 'expansive' or 'restrictive' the learning environment is (as discussed in Chapter 3), how much 'flex' there is within the clinical team to support peer-assisted learning and how much planning and preparation will be necessary including time for staff meetings, consultation, implementation and coaching training. The following activity can assist with the planning and implementation process.

Activity 3

Using the questions below, undertake an assessment of your clinical, therapeutic or practice area to determine readiness for peer-to-peer learning and use the results to decide which model of peer-assisted learning could be utilised with reference to Table 6.1.

- *How many staff are practice supervisors, assessors or educators?*
- *How many staff require practice supervisor, assessor or educator training?*
- *Which staff already have or could undertake coaching training?*
- *How do students experience interprofessional learning within the clinical area?*
- *What philosophy of care, management or therapy is in place?*
- *How is care delivered within the clinical or therapeutic area?*
- *How is the clinical area supported by the practice learning/education team?*
- *How is the clinical area supported by the university?*
- *What has characterised feedback given by learners who have completed a placement within the clinical or therapeutic area recently?*
- *What has characterised feedback given by practice supervisors/assessors/educators who have supported learners within the clinical/therapeutic area recently?*
- *What is the quality of the learning environment within the area?*
- *What has characterised feedback given by patients, clients, relatives and service users recently?*

Sustainable peer-assisted learning

It is not advisable to attempt to provide students with peer-assisted learning for the duration of the entire shift or even every day, particularly where senior students are being asked to 'take charge' and gain management experience. However, strategies that facilitate protected learning during the working day are particularly useful in promoting the welfare of students with special learning difficulties such as autism, where they are guaranteed an hour away from busy, noisy clinical environments to engage in peer-to-peer learning.

Protected learning time for students within busy clinical and therapeutic areas can be facilitated through the use of a 'power hour', where students are permitted to leave the practice area to complete negotiated learning activities linked to learning outcomes within their practice assessment documentation. The implementation of power hours can be a relatively sustainable first step in introducing peer-to-peer learning within clinical and therapeutic areas, particularly when staff are completing coaching training. Activities may include:

- Examination of medication charts to evaluate evidence of best practice in medicine management
- Creation of a poster presentation on a long-term condition, clinical or therapeutic procedure
- Risks and benefits analysis of a clinical investigation or operative procedure
- Appreciative inquiry relating to an episode of care, therapeutic management plan or patient intervention

- Review of the application, utilisation, application, effectiveness of an assessment model, approach or tool
- Facilitated student 'Schwartz-style round' where learners can explore the role of emotion arising from clinical and therapeutic intervention and engagement

Activity 4

Identify at least three learning activities that learners could complete and feedback to you as their practice supervisor/assessor when undertaking a 'power hour' within your clinical, therapeutic or practice area.

The role of the practice supervisor, assessor and educator is to ensure that peer learning opportunities are meaningful whilst ensuring that patient and client safety is not compromised. In order for students to hold conversations that matter, a structured approach can be introduced to ensure that protected learning times are productive and assist all learners to meet their learning outcomes. Here are some questions that can be used to structure learner dyad, triad or quad reflective meetings:

- *Where are you with … ?* [preparation for practice assessment, poster presentation, case study]
- *What do you think has just happened?* [within patient, client, staff interaction or episode of care]
- *What do you see?* [within this practice situation, clinical scenario, patient presentation, presenting illness]
- *What did you hear/observe?* [in this episode, as the patient deteriorated, during the assessment, case conference, tribunal, multi-disciplinary meeting]
- *What have you learnt?* [so far in this placement, from your practice supervisor/educator, during the visit]
- *What does it mean?* [for the patient, client, relative, informal carer, family]
- *How did you feel when … ?* [in relation to your beliefs, values, expectations, emotions]
- *What did you think would happen … ?* [to the patient, to the team, manager, organisation, service]
- *What might be the reason for that?* [episode, complaint, clinical presentation, diagnostic decision, management plan, investigation, referral]
- *What needs to happen next?* [for the patient, relative, team, department]
- *When will you know you have got it right?* [to be proficient, safe; to deliver effective, efficient care and demonstrate underpinning knowledge; to understand and place the values of the patient/client at the centre of care and management]
- *What do you need to pay attention to?* [communication, knowledge, understanding, knowing, skills, management, leadership, patient/staff advocacy, client enablement, empowerment]
- *What might you consider?* [alternate explanations, models, theories, explanatory frameworks, policies, legislation, assessment techniques, communicative actions, strategies, approaches, instructional techniques]
- *What would you do differently next time?* [if so why; if not why not; to whom and to what effect; based on an empirical approach, evidence, research; informed by best practice; drawing on personal knowledge]

- *What has been the muddiest point?* [that has confused, puzzled or surprised you]
- *If this were a story, what part would need to be told next?* [for the patient, client, service user, colleague, supervisor; team, department or clinical lead]

Reflective discussions can be facilitated online which affords students, apprentices and trainees with valuable skills in scheduling, facilitating and engaging with online meeting applications and programmes and the digital literacy and professional etiquette required.

Giving effective feedback

In the previous sections, we have explored the nature of 'conversations that matter' and how practice supervisors, assessors and educators can hold developmental reflective discussions to promote and facilitate transformational learning experiences for all. Additionally, we explored strategies for enabling students to engage in peer-to-peer learning that can provide learners with sufficient skills to become 'practice supervisor ready' at the point of graduation.

In this section, we will identify the key principles of giving effective feedback, which apply regardless of whether feedback is written or verbal. It is important that practice supervisors, assessors and educators reinforce the central messages and action points arising from meetings, in documentary form; not least as students can and do successfully appeal against assessment decisions. Appeals succeed when written feedback is poor, descriptive, opaque or simply absent from practice assessment documentation.

Activity 5

As Michael's practice assessor, you ask to examine his practice assessment document (PAD) to see how he has performed in undertaking patient assessment during his last placement. The following comment has been written in his PAD:
   'Michael performed his physical A-E patient assessment well'

1   To what extent does this written feedback assist both Michael and you as his practice assessor to get a sense of his performance and level of proficiency in the area of patient assessment?
2   What might be the implications of this feedback for practice supervisors and their ability to delegate and ensure Michael can safely participate in the assessment of patients?

Michael does not know how well he has actually performed. He does not know what areas need further development and why. The giver of the feedback has not described or evaluated the nature of Michael's performance including the accuracy, quality or effectiveness of the assessment, including the clinical implications. The conduct of the assessment and the outcome have not been differentiated.

Boud and Molloy (2013) argue that within professional environments there is a requirement to give feedback that not only engages the learner but enables them to start to come to judgements about their own performance. This process is known as 'Mark 2' feedback as the learner is in effect marking their own work, in addition to the practice supervisor, assessor and educator coming to a judgement regarding the learner's performance against proficiencies, competencies and recognised standards of work. Another characteristic of Mark 2 feedback is that it is always future referenced or forward facing, where the feedback giver points the learner to further practice learning opportunities, particularly when the performance has been deemed unsafe or sub-optimal within one occasion. This 'feed-forward' strategy ensures that the learner can contextualise their feedback as a journey of personal growth and development.

Managing emotions

Students, apprentices and learners should always be forewarned by their practice assessor, supervisor or educator that they are to receive feedback. Similarly, learners appreciate being asked to prepare for periods of questioning that enable the supervisor, assessor or educator to measure their current knowledge and under-standing. 'Cold calling', where students are put 'on the spot' and subjected to unexpected or lengthy questioning, may be experienced as intimidating or even perceived as bullying, even though most students are aware that being able to 'think on one's feet' is a professional necessity. Naturally, when feedback is provided to a student following an assessment of their performance, the learner may respond to adverse feedback in a negatively emotional or angry manner; particularly if the less than positive feedback is attached to a high stake's summative assessment. Whilst the practice supervisor, assessor and educator are accountable for their assessment decision-making, a non-judgemental approach where language is carefully chosen and attended to is preferable to feedback that the student may perceive as being incontestable, which in turn closes down the opportunity for a two-way discussion. Therefore, the practice supervisor, assessor or educator need to utilise their judgement to facilitate a discursive approach by giving feedback that is non-evaluative (avoiding the use of words such as 'good' or 'bad'), by focusing on the who, what, where, when, why and how of the performance. Whilst it is tempting to describe a student's practice as 'good', the receipt of such an affirmation may inadvertently discourage the learner to engage in a qualitative consideration of their own practice. In contrast, the supervisor, assessor or educator should facilitate a discussion that reflects on the performance of the learner through a structured discursive approach that Boud and Molloy (2013) suggest includes:

1　Asking the student, apprentice or trainee to describe the procedure, intervention or practice that they have been observed completing.
2　Asking the learner to evaluate their own performance in terms of what went well and not so well.
3　The practice supervisor, assessor and educator providing objective feedback using examples based on what has been observed against proficiencies and standards of work.
4　The learner and supervisor agreeing on what the next steps are, including strategies and goals to recover, remediate, enhance, develop or improve the student's performance further and how this might, could or shall be achieved depending on the actual outcome of the assessment.

Preparing to give feedback

In addition to the learner being forewarned that they are to receive feedback, practice supervisors, assessors and educators need to prepare themselves ahead of a meeting with a student or apprentice to ensure that the meeting is productive and completed efficiently; not least as it is likely that the feedback will be given towards the end of the day or shift. The supervisor/assessor needs to ask themselves to what end is the feedback intended and will the feedback need to be shared, perhaps with a practice assessor ahead of a summative or final assessment. Students will be expecting their practice assessment documentation to be completed. Therefore, it is important that the practice supervisor, assessor or educator is sufficiently familiar with the document to identify which parts need to be written, which will need to contain the 'must and need to know' feedback, as opposed to the 'nice to know' feedback that can be delivered verbally. Within busy clinical, therapeutic practice environments the most appropriate physical location needs to be identified in order for the learner to feel safe and able to receive and absorb the feedback. As we have seen when considering the nature of coaching, the supervisor/assessor may be required to give feedback during the student's performance, particularly if the learner is being directly supervised undertaking an assessment, clinical procedure or using a piece of diagnostic or therapeutic equipment. In this scenario, the practice supervisor/assessor may deliver feedback via a flow of information rather than a discursive approach as would be more appropriate post-performance. Inclusive (encouraging) vocabulary rather than final or incontestable feedback will enable the learner to respond and encourage questioning on the part of the student to elicit clarification. Within any feedback situation it is critical that the practice supervisor, assessor or educator is aware of their non-verbal dynamics such as body language, as the student may misinterpret facial reactions which may negatively impact their performance.

Activity 6

Sarbjit has arranged to spend an observation day with you as she is interested in cancer care and wants to spend a day in the cancer centre where, as her practice supervisor, you are employed to give intravenous chemotherapy to day patients. Having asked her to identify her learning needs, Sarbjit shows you the following written feedback from her previous 'base placement':

'Sarbjit's communication skills need improvement.'

1   To what extent does the feedback enable Sarbjit to identify her learning needs when provided with a short placement experience?
2   What might be the implications of the feedback on your ability to engage Sarbjit in participatory learning during her day in the cancer centre?

Sarbjit has not been told what type (verbal or non-verbal) or aspect of her communication skills needs improving and how. No attempt has been made to describe how she has communicated, with whom and to what effect.

Written feedback

At the start of this section, the consequences of poor or inadequate completion of students' practice assessment documentation were outlined, particularly if a student fails in practice and decides to lodge an academic appeal via their approved educational institution. Practice assessors and educators that learn of the outcome of a successful appeal may feel frustrated and perceive that their assessment decision is not valued. However, academic appeals succeed because 'due process' has not been followed, where a student is able to demonstrate sufficient evidence that an assessment has not been conducted properly. Naturally, the burden of evidence rests upon what has or has not been documented within a practice assessment document and may include:

- Insufficient or lack of evidence to support the decision to fail a student undertaking a summative assessment;
- A student being directly prevented from booking initial or mid-point meetings in a timely manner sufficient for the student to pass their final summative assessment;
- Vague or opaque written feedback insufficient for a student to understand their areas for development following a fail at a mid-point meeting having failed their summative assessment;
- A vague or opaque action plan, or a plan lacking Specific, Measurable, Achievable, Relevant, and Time-Bound (SMART) goals, or the absence of an action plan following a fail at a mid-point meeting having subsequently failed their summative assessment;
- Insufficient time including rostered practice experience for the student to respond to an action plan ahead of their summative assessment;
- Insufficient or inconsistent support from a practice supervisor or practice educator sufficient for the student to be provided with an opportunity to practice and meet goals within their action plan ahead of a summative assessment;
- Inappropriate, offensive, subjective, biased written feedback within a practice assessment document that undermines or causes material distress to the student sufficient to affect their confidence and ability to practise;
- A lack of time or reasonable opportunity for the student to be assessed fairly, openly and transparently (outside of unexpected or reasonable clinical demands) due to the availability of the practice assessor or educator;
- A summative assessment decision which is made solely by an assessor who has not sought feedback from other appropriate members of the team, particularly where the proficiency or competency of the student or apprentice could have otherwise been confirmed;
- A failure of the practice assessor or educator to appropriately delegate the assessment of a particular proficiency or competency to another practice supervisor/assessor or educator (in line with professional regulatory body standard body guidance) that prevents a student from being assessed either formatively or summatively.

Obviously, the above list is not exhaustive, but it is important to remember that the person appointed within an approved educational institution to consider a student's appeal may not be a healthcare registrant and will make their decision based on the documentary evidence contained within the practice assessment documentation in line with the institution's regulations on assessment and processes for academic appeal.

Activity 7

As a community mental health nurse, you have just completed Jo's induction to her new placement. Whilst completing the checklist, you notice the following comment written during a formative episode of care assessment in Jo's last placement:

'Throughout the episode, Jo's care delivery was inefficient.'

1 What might be the outcome of her mid-point meeting and any practice assessment undertaken during the placement, if this feedback is ignored?
2 What is your responsibility, as the practice supervisor, to respond to this feedback?

The phrase 'care delivery' is opaque as no attempt has been made to describe what care was delivered, how it was delivered, why it was inefficient or an indication of what an acceptable standard of efficiency might be. The implications of Jo's care have not been made clear and for whom.

Using the right vocabulary

When undertaking a practice assessment, it is important that the practice supervisor, assessor or educator avoids making an assessment decision based on what is called 'norm referencing' where a student is assessed on what the assessor regards as the appropriate practice of a student based on their academic year, level of experience, previous placements or even their age and maturity. A fair, open and transparent practice assessment must only be conducted on the basis of the assessment guidance and structure contained within the practice assessment document. Similarly, the assessment strategy may feature a participatory learning approach where students, trainees and apprentices are expected to work towards the fulfilment of proficiencies ahead of a determined progression point (at the end of their academic year) based on a level of supervision which simultaneously will be expected to reduce ahead of their final summative assessment point. Most practice assessment strategies within health and social care do not include a grading system as it has been found that assessors feel pressured to give high grades leading to 'grade inflation' (Perry, 2015). Assessors may feel reluctant to give a student a lower grade than what has previously been awarded, whilst the student and assessor may be conscious that grades may determine the classification of the student's final award. There are arguments for and against the grading of clinical practice, although evidence suggests that the strongest deterrent is the use of grading rubrics that can be used for both formative and summative assessments. Rubrics should contain clearly defined performance criteria or elements, a detailed description of what performance looks like at each level (or grade) of proficiency and a rating scale that most commonly uses three or four points (Donaldson and Gray, 2012).

Activity 8

As a practice educator, you have just started to work with Nicky, who is on placement within an intermediate care team. Nicky has asked if he can accompany you on a community visit of a patient recently discharged from hospital following a fall. Nicky is keen to assess the patients balance by undertaking a gait assessment which features the

Berg balance score. You decide to check the competency framework within the practice assessment document so that you can assess Nicky appropriately and note the following comment from his last placement, where he spent some time with the falls team:

'When undertaking the Berg balance score, Nicky failed to maintain the patient's safety.'

1   To what extent does this feedback provide you with sufficient confidence to supervise Nicky during the assessment?
2   Would the feedback enable Nicky to recontextualise the skills and knowledge gained in the last placement within the intermediate care team?

There is no indication at what stage and how the patient's safety was not maintained and to what effect or what the implications might have been for the patient. The giver of the feedback has not commented on other aspects of completing the balance score, which may or not have been effective, efficient or accurate. Nicky would not know what level of competency he has, based on this feedback.

Once an assessment decision has been made and the practice supervisor, assessor, educator and student have held a discussion, written feedback can be recorded within the practice assessment documentation. As we have seen, it is important for the assessor to describe objectively the practice of the student as observed factually and to come to a judgement regarding the quality of their performance. Table 6.2 contains suggested words that can be used to describe the frequency or efficiency and level of practice in addition to making a qualitative assessment of performance. Assessment criteria has been adapted from the Common Placement Assessment Form created by the Chartered Society of Physiotherapy (CSP, 2021).

Activity 9

Chris is midway through his first year and is engaging well, both with participatory and opportunistic learning within the department. She is working hard on her medication management, but when questioned on anatomy and physiology in relation to presenting illness, struggles to demonstrate underpinning knowledge. You discuss this with her practice assessor, who agrees and shares that they have documented this observation within her practice assessment documentation.

On examination of the document, you read the following feedback:
'Chris needs to demonstrate a deeper knowledge of A&P.'

1   As Chris's nominated practice supervisor, what conversation needs to be held with the practice assessor to make sense of the feedback and support Chris, going forward?
2   What bearing might the feedback have if Chris were to fail her next practice assessment in this area and what might the implications be for the practice assessor?

Chris has not been told which aspects of anatomy and physiology need to be studied, why and to what effect. No reference has been made to a patient or clinical incident, which means that Chris would not be able to contextualise the feedback or begin to understand the consequences or clinical implications of not having sufficient knowledge.

Table 6.2 Choosing and using suitable vocabulary for written feedback

How often? FREQUENCY	How well? AT WHAT LEVEL	Typical grade	Assessment criteria (adapted from the CPAF (CSP, 2021))	How? QUALITY OF STUDENT'S PERFORMANCE
WORDS TO USE	WORDS TO USE			WORDS TO USE
CONSISTENTLY ALWAYS CONSTANTLY WITHOUT FAIL	EXCELLENT REALLY WELL EXEMPLARY SUPERB OUTSTANDING EXCEPTIONAL	A	Outstanding (90–100%): Consistently achieves without support Exceptional (80–89%): Achieves most of the time without support Excellent (70–79%): Appropriately and proactively seeks support to achieve	CALMLY CORRECTLY REGULARLY DELIBERATELY EASILY QUICKLY ENTHUSIASTICALLY EXPERTLY PERFECTLY PROMPTLY
GENERALLY USUALLY NORMALLY	WELL DEVELOPED CAPABLE PROFICIENT SKILLFUL EXPERT ADEPT VERY GOOD WELL COMMENDABLE	B	Very Good (60–69%): Appropriately seeks support to achieve	QUICKLY QUIETLY RAPIDLY REGULARLY RELIABLY STEADILY REPEATEDLY SUCCESSFULLY SKILFULLY THOUGHTFULLY
SOMETIMES OCCASIONALLY	MEETS REQUIRED STANDARD	C	Good (50–59%): Requires support to achieve	WELL EASILY CONCISELY

(Continued)

Table 6.2 (Continued)

How often? FREQUENCY	How well? AT WHAT LEVEL	Typical grade	Assessment criteria (adapted from the CPAF (CSP, 2021))	How? QUALITY OF STUDENT'S PERFORMANCE
RARELY INCONSISTEN-TLY BEGINS TO ONCE SELDOM INFREQUENTLY	SATISFACTORY ADEQUATE ACCEPTABLE BARELY MEETS THE REQUIRED STANDARD/ REASONABLE	D	Satisfactory (40–49%): Requires significant support to achieve	ACCURATELY SENSITIVELY RESPONSIBLY PROFESSIONALLY PRECISELY RELIABLY APPROPRIATELY
NEVER HAS NOT DEMONSTRA-TED DOES NOT DEMONSTR-ATE FAILS TO DEMONSTR-ATE	UNSATISFACTORY POOR INADEQUATE FAILS TO MEET REQUIRED STANDARD	E/FAIL	Fail (30–39%): Does not achieve despite feedback and support Fail (0–29%): Does not achieve despite significant feedback and support	

Perpetual proficiency

We discussed earlier the importance of students receiving forward-facing, future referenced or 'feed-forward' feedback, where the learner is given feedback that is situated in the future, where an assessor may point to opportunities to work with them or another supervisor/assessor to develop their practice further, utilising additional learning opportunities or appropriate episodes of care. This is particularly relevant where practice assessment documentation affords the student and apprentice of learner with multiple opportunities for their proficiencies to be re-assessed, particularly when moving from one clinical or therapeutic area to another, where a proficiency needs to be met in a slightly different way due to the clinical speciality, needs of clients or clinical acuity of patients. It is important for practice supervisors, assessors and educators to explain the concept of proficiency as a process of perpetuity, not least as all practitioners, therapists and clinicians are required to maintain their levels of proficiency in response to research, evidence and what constitutes best practice within ever-changing and super complex practice landscapes.

In summary, feedback is more effective when:

- There is a balance of comments that confirm good performance whilst emphasising improvement of performance in relation to standards of good work.
- Provides objective examples based on the observed practice of the student, where the practice supervisor, assessor or educator comments on aspects of work and the behaviour of the learner rather than them as a person or feedback characterised by 'broad brush' generalisations.
- Written and verbal feedback that is 'future referenced', where supervisors, assessors and educators seek to identify how improvements can be made, what strategies are required and asks the student to identify whether they are achievable.
- The feedback discussion ends with a summary that enables the practice supervisor, assessor or educator to check the shared understanding of both parties and encourage the learner to record the 'take-home' or 'takeaway' messages.

Activity 10

Max, a final-year occupational therapy student, has just received written feedback that contains the following sentence, which she finds puzzling:
'Leadership does not appear to be this student's forte.'

1 Max is afraid to seek clarification from the practice educator who provided the feedback. Why might this be so?
2 What might be the implications if Max is unable to recognise the significance of this feedback and to whom?

The feedback not only lacks specificity but is incontestable. No examples from practice have been provided and the giver of the feedback has conveyed an impression of absolute failure to the student. Again, no practice examples have been given to support the assertion.

Effective written and verbal feedback is contingent on both the learner and supervisor/assessor adopting a goal-setting approach, that focuses on performance (the how, what, where, when, why and whom of patient/client care) and the student determining further steps to achieve their goals which may include the enhancement of what has already been identified as safe, effective, efficient practice with sufficient underpinning knowledge.

The role of emotion for the supervisor/assessor

In this chapter, we have explored the nature of transformational learning and how practice supervisors, assessors and educators can engage in meaningful conversations with students, whilst facilitating peer-to-peer learning opportunities to enable them to have conversations that matter. We have identified the importance of being able to give effective feedback to a range of learners and why it is important to be accountable for the assessment decisions made. In Chapter 2, we saw that professional regulatory standards bodies such as the Nursing and Midwifery Council (NMC) and other bodies such as the College of Operating Department Practitioners (CODP) have introduced standards to ensure that the assessment and support of students is undertaken through a separation of the roles of practice supervisor and assessor. However, whilst this strategy may help to enhance the reliability of assessment practice (Duffy, 2004), assessors and supervisors continue to experience a considerable range of emotions when supporting, assessing and failing students (Finch and Taylor, 2013; Larocque and Luhanga, 2013). Therefore, it is important that practice supervisors, assessors and educators engage in personal reflection to uncover thoughts and feelings and make sense of strong emotions associated with the support of a student who may have failed in practice; not least as the supervisor/assessor needs to be sure that the student has failed by their own hand and not been consciously or inadvertently disadvantaged by factors associated with the quality of the practice, clinical, therapeutic or working environment. Scott and Spouse (2013) suggest that in order to reflect on a difficult event, the recognition and acknowledgement of feelings is necessary before sense-making can occur and highlight that practice supervisors and educators need to be able to recognise when an experience has consciously or unconsciously reminded them of other students or complex situations with learners.

Values-based reflection

Whilst there is a myriad of different reflective models available, the Me, My, More, Must model (Wareing, 2017) facilitates reflection from the perspective of examining the impact of professional values on practice. The model (see Table 6.3) was designed to help learners consider who they are and what impact their values might have before a description of the particular experience, situation or incident. As stated at the beginning of this chapter, the central premise of the model is that learning within practice and the workplace is a profoundly lived experience that requires educators to identify, analyse and make sense of the impact of their values in order to become the educationalist that they aspire to be.

Most approved educational institutions, such as universities, provide debriefing or appreciative inquiry meetings for practice supervisors, assessors and educators who have

Table 6.3 Values-based reflection

Stages	Prompts
Me	Which values are important to me as a learner in the workplace?
	What feelings have I experienced since supporting my learner?
	What has enabled me to be able to practise effectively as an educator?
My	What values underpin my role as a supervisor/assessor/educator?
	How have my feelings changed during the experience?
	What concerns do I have regarding myself?
	To what extent were my values challenged as a result of supervising/assessing my learner?
More	What questions have been generated from this experience?
	What do I need more of in order to continue to support learners?
	What evidence do I want to see more of in order for me to be able assess my learner in a fair, open and transparent way?
Must	What must I do to address my learning goals?
	What values must I explore to be able to support learners more effectively?
	What must you do in order for me to become the educator that I wish to become?

experienced challenging, complex, difficult or upsetting experiences with students, particularly where they have had to fail a student; perhaps for the first time. Completing a piece of written reflection is a useful strategy for making sense of such an experience and as we saw earlier, is useful for understanding emotion and obtaining support from academic staff to review the assessment process, documentation, the quality of written feedback and identify personal learning points to develop insight and confidence.

Summary

In this chapter, we have seen the critical importance of the role of practice supervisors, assessors and educators in providing and evaluating learning experiences from the perspective of the extent to which they are transformational for the learner. The nature of communicative action was characterised by the need for learners to engage in conversations that matter, not only with their supervisors and assessors, but through peer-to-peer learning. Protected learning time or specific models such using a coaching and peer-assisted learning approach require careful selection, coaching training, placement preparation and implementation. Coaching techniques such as questioning can be adopted by students within a range of configurations, which afford senior students with opportunities for management, leadership and the facilitation of learning. Giving effective feedback is a process that can instil an 'inner dialogue' sufficient for the student to develop reflective, developmental learning disposition that can serve their entire professional life. The feedback giver needs to attend to the words, vocabulary and language used and consider a range of contextual factors to minimise the effect of negative emotional responses and labour, whilst recognising that the attainment of proficient practice is a perpetual process. Finally, in accordance with the need for students to be assessed on their professional values, it was argued that practice supervisors, assessors and educators can utilise experiences with students, apprentices and learners to engage in values-based reflection to enhance their capabilities and effectiveness and to become the educator that they aspire to be.

References

Boud, D, Molloy, E (eds) (2013) *Feedback in higher and professional education: Understanding it and doing it well*. London: Routledge.

Claridge, MT, Lewis, T (2005) *Coaching for effective learning: A practical guide for teachers in healthcare*. London: Routledge.

CSP (2021) *Common placement assessment form (CPAF)*. London: Chartered Society of Physiotherapy. https://www.csp.org.uk/professional-clinical/practice-based-learning/cpaf

Donaldson, JH, Gray, M (2012) 'Systematic review of grading practice: Is there evidence of grade inflation?' *Nurse Education in Practice*, 12 (2), pp. 101–114, 10.1016/j.nepr.2011.10.007

Duffy, K (2004) *Failing Students: A qualitative study of factors that influence the decisions regarding assessment of students' competence in practice*. London: NMC.

Finch, J, Taylor, I (2013) 'Failure to fail? Practice educators' emotional experiences of assessing failing social work students', *Social Work Education*, 32(2), pp. 244–258, 10.1080/02615479.2012.720250

Foster-Turner, J (2006) *Coaching and mentoring in health and social care: The essential manual for professionals and organisations*. Abingdon: Radcliffe Press.

Illeris, K (2014) *Transformative learning and identity*. London: Routledge.

Larocque, S, Luhanga, FL (2013) 'Exploring the issue of failure to fail in a nursing program', *International Journal of Nursing Education Scholarship*, 10(1), pp. 1–8.

Perry, V (2015) 'Grade inflation in the assessment of clinical practice', *Journal of Pedagogic Practice*, 5 (3), pp. 3–8, https://uobrep.openrepository.com/bitstream/handle/10547/584270/224-606-1-PB.pdf?sequence=1&isAllowed=y

Raelin, JA (2008) *Work-based learning: Bridging knowledge and action in the workplace*. Hoboken, NJ: Jossey-Bass.

Schön, D (1991) *The reflective practitioner: How professionals think in action*. New York: Taylor & Francis.

Scott, I, Spouse, J (2013) *Practice-based learning in nursing, health and social care: Mentorship, facilitation and supervision*. Oxford, Wiley-Blackwell.

Wareing, M (2017) 'Me, my, more, must: A values-based model of reflection', *Reflective Practice, International and Multidisciplinary Perspectives*, 18, pp. 268–279, https://www.tandfonline.com/doi/abs/10.1080/14623943.2016.1269002

Wareing, M, Green, H, Burden, B, Burns, S, Beckwith, MAR, Mhlanga, F, Mann, B (2018) 'Coaching and peer assisted learning (C-PAL) – The mental health nursing experience: A qualitative evaluation', *Journal of Psychiatric & Mental Health Nursing*, 25, pp. 486–495, https://onlinelibrary.wiley.com/doi/abs/10.1111/jpm.12493

Chapter 7

Supporting health, well-being and promoting inclusivity

Mark Wareing and Adrienne Sharples

By the end of this chapter, you will be able to:

1 Identify at least four signifiers of a student in difficulty.
2 Describe at least four key requirements of an action plan.
3 Critically analyse the role of the educator in promoting wellbeing within the learning environment for all.
4 Explore the role of the educator as a guardian of inclusive learning.

Introduction

The focus of this chapter will be on supporting practice supervisors, educators and assessors to recognise and support students in difficulty and, where appropriate, use strategies such as mediation and appreciative inquiry to facilitate difficult conversations and resolve conflict and incivility. The role of action planning in remediating and developing students and apprentices will be promoted as a non-punitive, purposeful approach to the remediation and enhancement of practice performance. Additionally, the critical importance of student, apprentice and learner wellbeing will be examined within the context of recognising and celebrating difference within practice learning settings that are safe, compassionate and inclusive.

Mental health and wellbeing of learners

Those hoping to join the 'helping professions' are often motivated by a wish to care and provide a contribution to their community (Wareing et al., 2024). Although working in a health and social care setting can be emotionally rewarding, this work can contribute to staff experiencing mental health issues such as stress, anxiety and depression at rates often higher than other occupational sectors (Health and Safety Executive, 2022). The demands of practising during the COVID-19 pandemic presented a mixed picture in terms of impact on mental health and general wellbeing. In some health and social care sectors, despite this stressful situation, staff experienced better outcomes, including improved career satisfaction, quality of working life and mental wellbeing (McFadden et al., 2022). In others, the pandemic played a part in practice staff experiencing poorer mental health (Couper et al., 2022; Lamb et al., 2022).

It is important to remember that while students may not be in practice full time, they also experience challenges during their course that may contribute to poorer mental

DOI: 10.4324/9781003358602-7

health and wellbeing. Stressors may stem from personal circumstances including meeting caring demands or having to take paid employment alongside the course. Additionally, there are stressors associated with the academic or practice aspect of training. For example, applying theory to practical situations can often lead to feelings of a lack of preparedness when working with service users (King-Okoye and Arber, 2014; Wallace et al., 2015). Academic stressors include the intellectual and time demands associated with the course, along with the volume of work and meeting academic demands whilst out in practice (e.g. Mandy et al., 2006; Hamshire et al., 2013).

In the first instance, practice supervisors, assessors and educators can help their students' wellbeing by ensuring they are welcomed and orientated within the practice area and regularly checking that they feel that they 'belong' within the practice area. Indeed, this type of support cannot be under estimated as the feeling of belonging in practice can influence whether students feel they have someone they can turn to when experiencing problems, and their intent to continue in the profession after graduation (Levett-Jones and Lathlean, 2009a; 2009b; Borrott et al., 2016). One way to foster a sense of belonging in students is to offer social support with aim of positively influencing mental wellbeing and building self-esteem and resilience (e.g. Hou et al., 2020). Social support can be provided in a number of ways, including emotional (compassion and caring), instrumental (use of time and resources), appraisal (self-evaluation and positive feedback) and informational (sharing information). It is essential that practice staff are aware of the different ways that support can be provided to students through a range of opportunities within the practice area.

We all have individual needs, so it is important to remember when supporting learners in practice to regularly 'check in' with them to assess whether they are getting their individual needs met. There is some evidence that an individual's personality and their 'personal resources', such as coping mechanisms, resilience and self-efficacy, will influence their need to belong, need for support and how they experience stressors within practice. In order to support students from minoritized backgrounds, it is important to build cultural competence to help meet individual needs. Some minority students may experience lowered feelings of belonging in practice due to entering an unwelcoming atmosphere where they feel disliked by staff, or have difficulty in finding staff that share their professional and personal values (Sedgwick et al., 2014). In order to deliver effective support for students from different backgrounds, practice staff need to have completed the equality, diversity and inclusivity (EDI) training offered within their workplace. Additionally, practice supervisors, assessors and educators can introduce students and apprentices to workplace societies with an EDI focus, or connect with staff from a similar background to the learner so that they have an ally or 'buddy'.

Activity I

Think about an episode from your life span where you struggled as a learner or experienced a learning disappointment; this could be an examination, practicum or practice-based assessment that you found puzzling or where the outcome was not what you expected.

1   What emotions and feelings made it a vivid experience?
2   Who was involved and what were their roles and responsibilities?

3   How was the incident resolved and by whom?
4   What impact did the experience have on your confidence as a learner?

Understanding the needs of the failing learner

Failing an examination, assignment or practical assessment can be a devastating experience for learners and is likely to be characterised by embarrassment, disappointment and anxiety, as the consequences of the failure are processed and the implications realised. Within an adult learning setting, the experience of academic or practice failure may be closely associated with the learning identity of the student (Wojecki, 2016), which may be deeply associated with an experience perhaps decades earlier (Askham, 2008), having an impact on the agency of the learner (Mercer, 2007; Biesta and Tedder, 2016) and their ability to move forward. If a student experienced a traditional form of schooling characterised by 'front-loaded' teaching and regular formal testing, their perception of what is regarded as an acceptable performance may be artificially high and this may present particular challenges when a student is being graded in practice, let alone failed in an assessment. Within some cultures, academic failure (Najimi *et al.*, 2013; Ajjawi, 2020) may be seen as shameful or dishonourable, particularly if a young learner is being supported by parents or family and has moved overseas to undertake study where entrance to a profession is highly prized. Conversely, a mature student may struggle with failure if they are working hard to be a role model before their own offspring and are active in encouraging their educational attainment (Wainwright and Marandet, 2010).

In earlier chapters, we have looked at the role of the practice supervisor and educator in enabling the student, learner or apprentice to make sense of the 'what, where, when, how, why and whom' of their practice performance. Whilst it may not always be the case, a learner may demonstrate sub-optimal care, practice and proficiency prior to formative or summative assessment, which will require the practice supervisor/educator to review not only the performance of the learner, but decide whether the style and level of supervisory support and intervention is appropriate to maintain patient and client safety in addition to the provision of guided learning, instruction and practice teaching. Whilst a practice supervisor or assessor may have been alerted to the performance of the learner by another practitioner, member of staff, patient, client or service user, it is critical that a holistic assessment is undertaken of the immediate needs and associated behaviours of the student who should be regarded as a learner in difficulty.

Identifying the learner in difficulty

The Common Placement Assessment Form (CSP, 2021) encourages practice educators to engage in a dialogue with learners to ensure that there is an awareness of factors that may be causing difficulties for students and apprentices. These factors include:

- Concerns about risk of discrimination linked to protected characteristics (age, disability, gender reassignment, race, religion or belief, sex, sexual orientation, marriage and civil partnership and pregnancy and maternity);
- Concerns regarding accessibility/access to reasonable adjustments;

- Social or family circumstances such as living environment, caring responsibilities or travel issues;
- Health or wellbeing issues relating to physical and/or mental health;
- Financial issues such as travel costs or access;
- Religious or cultural beliefs, values or practices;
- Previous problems encountered during placements;
- Previous experiences such as bereavement, personal or family health or wellbeing issues that may be relevant to how the learner experiences the placement setting.

A practice supervisor, educator or assessor needs to undertake a holistic assessment in order to identify:

1 What behaviour or practice has actually been observed and by whom; where, when, how frequent and to what effect.
2 Whether the behaviour or practice includes communication (either written, verbal, electronic, non-verbal) and the impact of the communicative actions, for whom and to what effect.
3 The relationship between the observed behaviour or practice against accepted standards of work or regulatory standard professional body standards or codes.
4 To what extent the observed behaviour or practice render the student, apprentice or learner's performance proficient or even inept, inexpert, unsafe and incompetent.
5 To what extent the student, apprentice or learner is experiencing emotional stress, what these stressors are and the extent to which they may or may not be outside of their control.
6 If the student has a previously undisclosed special learning need or disability.
7 Whether the learner experienced a recent upsetting or traumatic event within the clinical, therapeutic or practice environment associated with the care or loss of a patient, client or service user.
8 Whether the student, learner or apprentice has experienced moral distress or moral injury arising from an episode of care or event that was incongruent with their values, beliefs or moral framework.
9 The extent to which the student or apprentice has insight into the quality of their performance, practice, effect, significance and implications of their behaviour and on whom.
10 The influence of factors such as the safety of the practice environment; the expansiveness of the learning environment; the quality of the working environment including staff levels, skill mix, patient/client and service user acuity; ratio of student to practice supervisor/educator and extent of direct, indirect and arm's-length supervision.

Whilst there is never a single approach for managing a student in difficulty, a practice supervisor or educator needs to feel sufficiently confident to hold an initial informal meeting with the student or apprentice to share their concerns by objectively exploring the observed practice and behaviour of the student in a factual manner, with reference to dates, days, times, those present and if necessary the actual words spoken. If a practice supervisor/educator is new to their role or inexperienced in holding difficult conversations with students and apprentices, they may wish to seek support from the student's practice assessor, another practice supervisor/educator or contact the student's university to ask if a link lecturer/tutor could attend the meeting to ensure that all parties are appropriately supported and that the focus of the meeting is on the needs of the learner.

If a student, apprentice or learner's practice or behaviour is identified as unsafe and their professional conduct falls below the standard required by professional standard regulatory body published standards and codes, a practice supervisor, educator or practice assessor may decide to formally report the student to the university in accordance with the institution's cause for concern or fitness to practice policy and procedure. However, it must be noted that a cause for concern can also be used as a formal mechanism for the reporting of a welfare concern rather than an action orientated to a disciplinary process. In such a case, it is incumbent upon the person completing the cause for concern report to explain this to the student or apprentice, to avert them from regarding the action as punitive.

Activity 2

What does the term 'cause for concern' mean to you in the context of:

- Patient, client or service user experience?
- Patient, client or service user safety, wellbeing and safeguarding?
- Students, apprentices and trainees?

Inevitably, the phrase 'cause for concern' may be associated with raising a concern in practice arising from a patient/client safety or safeguarding issue, or the observation of a practitioner's behaviour that leads to a discussion relating to their professional values and conduct. It is important to acknowledge that a cause for concern report relating to a particular student or apprentice may describe behaviours relating to a constellation of factors associated with the immediate workplace and relationships between staff leading to incivility; all of which may be deeply associated with the welfare of a learner and their ability to function within a placement or practice learning experience.

Making sense of cause for concern

In the previous section, we saw that the raising of a cause for concern to a learner's university may relate simply to a concern for their welfare, rather than as a result of their practice being unsafe or their behaviour and conduct falling short of regulatory body standards or a code. A student in difficulty may be identified as a cause for concern regarding their welfare if:

- They appear pre-occupied with matters outside of the practice or placement setting such as childcare, housing, debt, addiction, fulfilling informal care or sustaining an income sufficient for them to continue their studies.
- They arrive on placement late or appear tired, withdrawn, tearful or are uncharacteristically quiet or are isolating themselves.

- Travel to and from the placement or the availability of public transport becomes difficult, arduous or places the student at risk sufficient to threaten attendance, engagement or successful completion of the placement.
- A student is behind with their clinical hours, academic study, preparation of assignments, revision for examinations or objective structured clinical examinations (OSCEs).
- An apprentice is struggling to be recognised as a learner in their own right, in contrast to other students.
- An apprentice or student is struggling to balance working with learning.
- A student or apprentice lacks confidence in arranging or initiating their own learning experiences, is unable to articulate their learning needs, lacks sufficient confidence in arranging mid-point and final formative/summative practice assessments and requesting the completion of their practice assessment documentation in a timely manner.
- A learner struggles to engage in participatory learning sufficient for their level of practice.
- A student's personally held beliefs and values are creating or have the potential to create a barrier to the delivery of safe and effective care of patients, clients and service users.

Fitness to practice

Whilst this list is not exhaustive, it must be noted that all of the above areas can be effectively managed by practice supervisors, educators and assessors, although when a particularly serious, unlawful, patient safety or safeguarding incident occurs, it is incumbent on senior practice partners to contact the university and consider an immediate suspension of the student's placement, leading to a referral to the Fitness to Practice committee or panel. In such a situation, an investigating officer for the university will be appointed to undertake a formal investigation, although it would not be permissible for this to be concurrent with an investigation involving the police. Ordinarily, in accordance with the university's Fitness to Practice policy, a student or apprentice subject to a Fitness to Practice case, will be formally interviewed and may attend with a friend or family member for support only. The investigating officer will also be required to interview all other parties and triangulate their findings, alongside a timeline of events with their conclusions and map recommendations against the relevant professional standard regulatory body code or standards. The Fitness to Practice panel will be chaired by a senior academic manager (usually a head of school, associate or executive dean), comprised of practice partners, an internal academic member of staff and at least one person who holds current registration with the professional regulatory body matched to the student's programme of study. The format of the Fitness to Practice panel usually involves a presentation of the investigating officers' key findings (within their written report), an opportunity for the panel to question both the investigating officer and student and time for the panel to deliberate and if possible, agree on a judgement that is normally disclosed to the student at a later date. Students may appeal against the judgement of the Fitness to Practice panel and should be strongly advised to seek impartial advice and support from the university's student services, students' union or trade union, throughout the process.

Activity 3

Dom is a final-year pre-registration adult nursing student who is midway through a placement in a day surgery unit (DSU) within a general hospital. His previous placements have included general medicine, a spinal unit, an adult community healthcare team and a hospice. Mike and Svetlana, Dom's practice supervisor and assessor, meet to discuss his progress ahead of the mid-point formative assessment scheduled during his 12-week placement. Mike shares that Dom has settled well into the clinical area, but is struggling to retain information relating to the pre-operative preparation of patients for a range of elective procedures. Additionally, Dom's knowledge and understanding of analgesics is poor. Svetlana shared a concern from another practice supervisor, Clara, that on several occasions Dom has become defensive and agitated when asked to describe and evaluate his performance, having been supervised undertaking clinical procedures such as wound care or safely preparing patients for discharge.

1   How should Svetlana and Mike prepare Dom for his mid-point formative assessment?
2   What are the implications of Dom's current performance in relation to the likely outcome of his mid-point assessment?
3   What would the implications be if Dom were to pass his mid-point assessment ahead of being assessed summatively, either in this or his final placement?
4   What actions and interventions might Svetlana and Mike consider in order to complete the mid-point assessment and support the student for the remainder of the placement?

Action planning

It is clear within the last vignette that Svetlana and Mike need to make Dom aware of their concerns relating to his performance ahead of the mid-point assessment, so that the assessment follows the principal of 'no surprises'. This can be achieved by ensuring that there is written feedback within the practice assessment documentation that is shared with Dom and can be cited during the mid-point meeting. If Dom were to pass his mid-point assessment based on being given the 'benefit of the doubt', it would be difficult for his practice assessor to justify failing him as Dom may not be aware that his performance is sub-optimal, particularly if Svetlana and Mike have not placed him on an action plan that clearly details his areas of development against the assessment criteria and proficiencies. Once an action plan is written, Dom can meet with Svetlana to review his progress and be given sufficient time and opportunity to practice and demonstrate improvement, sufficient for him to be prepared for his final summative assessment with Mike, who in turn will be required to obtain feedback from Svetlana and other practice supervisors (in accordance with the NMC SSSA, 2023) to complete a fair, open, transparent final assessment of Dom in accordance with the assessment criteria and requirements of the practice assessment documenta- tion. Again, involving a link lecturer from the university at the mid-point and final assessment ensures that all parties are supported, particularly if the student is to be failed. not least to ensure that the practice assessor is able to reach an assessment decision that is accountable on the basis of the written evidence contained within the practice assessment document.

Activity 4

Dom negotiates a time for Svetlana and Mike to complete his mid-point assessment, which takes place off the day surgery unit. In preparation for the meeting, Mike forewarns Dom that he is concerned that he is not demonstrating sufficient underpinning knowledge in order to pass his medicines management assessment that is scheduled for his next and final placement and that this will need to be discussed alongside other areas for development at the mid-point meeting. Dom arrives at the meeting looking anxious and when Svetlana shares Clara's experience where Dom was defensive and became agitated when asked to evaluate his performance changing a dressing, Dom highlights the range of proficiencies that have been signed off relating to wound care in previous placements. He also cites his lack of recent acute experience as a factor relating to his current performance. When Svetlana explains that Dom is not able to pass his mid-point assessment and requires an action plan, Dom becomes tearful and says, 'Will me being put on report mean I will be kicked off the course if I fail this placement?'
    Imagine that you are Svetlana:

1   How would you explain the purpose of the action plan to Dom?
2   What sources of evidence are needed to identify Dom's learning and development needs?
3   What external factors might explain Dom's response to being informed of the need of an action plan?
4   What does Dom need to understand regarding the assessment of his proficiency?
5   How might Dom's learning preferences be considered to enable him to engage more effectively in participatory and opportunistic learning?

Svetlana needs to explain to Dom that the primary purpose of an action plan is developmental, to enable him to be actively involved in the identification of his learning needs, based on observed examples from practice, which are evaluated against standards of work in accordance with the NMC (2023) code and proficiencies contained within his practice assessment document. An action plan is not punitive, but supportive, but should include goals that are achievable within the timeframe between the mid-point and final summative assessment. Svetlana may need to explore with Dom the background to his expressed emotions; in particular, his perception that being on an action plan renders his status as a student in jeopardy. Dom may not be aware that the NMC SSSA (2023) standards require practice assessors to make an assessment decision by gathering written and verbal evidence from other practice supervisors and that such a process should not be used, seen or regarded as a 'conspiracy to fail'. Additionally, Dom needs to understand that whilst he may have been assessed as proficient in previous placements, it is permissible for proficiencies to be re-assessed within different contexts to ensure that his skills do not fade and to ensure that practice proficiency is recontextualised against local standards of work pertinent to the clinical speciality and particular needs of the patient group. Lastly, the early identification of enablers and any barriers to learning will ensure that Dom's developmental needs are tailored to his preferred style of learning, which, if identified, will enable Svetlana and Mike to match learning opportunities to activities that Dom can participate in, to meet his action plan.

Inclusive practice learning

In Chapter 1, we were introduced to the notion of compassionate practice learning environments, which are based on a strategic commitment to ensuring that students, apprentices and trainees are enabled to learn through inclusive as well as supportive approaches. Inclusive and compassionate practice learning environments seek to ensure that learners are not prevented from learning and practicing due to protected characteristics, such as age, disability, ethnicity, nationality, sexuality, gender, pregnancy, religious belief, being married or in a civil partnership; or personal characteristics such as their social background or status as a student, apprentice or by being regarded as 'unqualified'.

Nixon (2019, p. 2) argues that there ' … are norms, patterns and structures in society that work for or against certain groups of people, which are unrelated to their individual merit or behaviour … unfair social structures have profound effects on health, producing inequities in morbidity and mortality'. Nixon describes the nature of privilege using the metaphor of a coin, which represents the system of inequality either taken or received by an individual whose lived experience is categorised by either side of the coin. The 'face' or top the coin represents the privileged, where a person has unearned advantages because of who they happen to be, in contrast to the 'back' or bottom of the coin where a person has unearned disadvantages because of who they happen to be. The coin represents the lived experiences of privilege in comparison to the experience of oppression.

Students and apprentices from minoritized backgrounds may be disadvantaged by their accent, if English is not their first language or if practice staff perceive that their name is unfamiliar or if they are treated differently for being minoritized on the basis of gender.

Activity 5

Think about your position as a practice supervisor, assessor or educator:

1   To what extent does your professional, social, ethnic or cultural background render particular personal advantage? What advantages might they be?
2   To what extent might your professional, social, ethnic or cultural background reflect the lived experience of your students or apprentices?
3   What experiences have you had relating to language that you would now perceive as examples of un-inclusive practices.

Nixon (2019) concludes that the key task for people is to understand that there is a coin, that it has two sides and that they may occupy the position of unearned advantage. Developing the capacity to ask and answer questions such as' *In which ways did I benefit from my privilege today?'* and *"In what ways did my actions today reflect and thereby reinforce my privilege?'* is necessary to ensure that students, apprentices and learners are not systemically disadvantaged, oppressed or discriminated against. Whilst it is recognised that people on the top of the coin did not ask for their unearned advantage, Nixon argues that people are rarely on the top of the coin because of merit or worth (commonly referred to as meritocracy).

'Rather, they are there, by definition, because they happen to be able-bodied, settlers, white, straight, cisgender, or other aspects of their social identity that they did not choose, but which nonetheless align with historic planes of domination and subordination' (Nixon, 2019, p. 5). We have seen that belongingness is strongly related to the extent to which students and apprentices are able to engage successfully in all forms of participatory and opportunistic learning. The cultural, social and ethnic background of learners as well as emotional factors play a key part in the extent to which a practice learning environment can be said to be truly inclusive.

You may have found the completion of Activity 5 both challenging and uncomfortable, particularly if like the writers of this chapter you recognise that you possess characteristics which render privilege; both within your professional and educational role or if you were reminded of personal characteristic (again like the authors!) that have resulted in discrimination.

Nixon (2019) asserts the need for the practice of critical allyship to dismantle inequality and re-orientate practice professional perspectives from helping the less fortunate through the use of expertise for the benefit of marginalised communities towards a range of personal commitment that includes:

- Seeking to understand your role in upholding systems of oppression that create inequality;
- Learning from the expertise of and working in solidarity with historically marginalised groups to help understand and take action on systems of inequality;
- Working to build insight among others in positions of privilege and mobilizing in collective action under the leadership of people 'on the bottom of the coin'.

(Nixon, 2019, p. 8)

Hammond et al.'s (2019) study into the lived experiences of physiotherapy students from a Black, Asian or minority ethnic (BAME) background revealed that participants experienced being an 'outsider' in what was perceived as a profession of white dominance in comparison to other health profession courses. Students' sense of belongingness was contingent on placing value on specific characteristics such as being extrovert and proactive, which at times would be in conflict with their racial/cultural backgrounds. As a consequence, students worked harder to demonstrate these characteristics when they felt disadvantaged.

Helpful and less helpful language

It is beyond the scope of this chapter to explore anti-discriminatory and anti-oppressive practice in great detail, but attending to the content and quality of conversation through the use of language is a critical feature of practising as a supervisor, assessor or educator in a compassionate and inclusive manner. Unhelpful language includes words and phrases that may 'trigger' an adverse response in the student or apprentice and is usually due to an implied judgement in the language or how it has been interpreted by the 'receiver'. Students and apprentices may become defensive, feel shut off from the conversation or begin to feel negative emotions such as anger or frustration. This type of unhelpful language is best avoided, particularly when holding a 'conversation that matters' (as discussed in Chapter 6) or a difficult conversation with a student or apprentices in difficulty, as discussed earlier in this chapter. There are several categories of unhelpful language to be aware of (Grimsley, 2010; Gillen, 2008).

Judgemental language is when phrases involve a negative judgement about a learner. The judgement may be direct or 'sneaky' in that the supervisor, assessor or educator does not take direct ownership of their judgement. This kind of language is likely to put the student or apprentice of the message in a defensive mode and cause an escalation of resistance and negative emotion.

Moralistic judgements may include:

"If you were not so busy ... ."

"If you actually listened to what I had said ..."

'Sneaky' judgements may include:

"It is obvious you cannot do this on your own ..."

"It's not appropriate ..."

"It's nonsense to think like that ..."

Parental language is autocratic and suggests that the supervisor, assessor or educator is powerful and superior. Students and apprentices may feel pushed back and disrespected, leading to an absence of mutual respect, learning or understanding.

Parental language includes:

"You must remember to ..."

"You ought, cannot, should ..."

An alternative strategy might be:

"Have you tried to ..."

"I would prefer you to ..."

Mind-reading language implies that you know either what the other person is thinking or what they are going to do and is based on assumptions held by the supervisor, assessor or educator that are more likely not true. Mind-reading should be distinguished from paraphrasing what a student or apprentice has said. Summarising what has been shared is actually a legitimate form of active listening, commonly used within coaching conversations, as discussed in Chapters 4 and 6. Examples of mind-reading might be:

"What you do not seem to realise is that ..."

"What you have clearly forgotten is that ..."

"But what you are actually saying is ..."

Irritator language is when words and phrases are used by supervisors, assessors and educators to strengthen their message or instructions. 'Irritator' language is characterised by saying the opposite of the truth, where the student or apprentice may perceive the opposite of what has been said rendering the conversation unconstructive. Examples might be:

> *"With all due respect"* [The supervisor, assessor, educator does not respect the learner as an insult is on its way!]

> *"I hear what you are saying"* [There is no intention of listening to what the learner has to say].

> *"Okay, let's be realistic here"* [Implies the student or apprentice has been completely unrealistic].

Formal language is unnecessarily rigid rather than conversational and may include jargon, abbreviations or acronyms, which conveys authority over the learner and is therefore disrespectful and un-inclusive.
Examples include:

> *"At this moment in time …"*

> *"In the fulness of time…"*

> *"Furthermore … henceforth …"*

> *"The completion of the IPR needs to be undertaken PDQ if we are to avoid any brick bats from HR"*

> *"Let us not be under any illusion that …"*

Activity 6

In Chapter 3, we looked at the importance of welcoming students and apprentices through induction and one-to-one meetings. What role do you have as a practice supervisor, assessor and educator in ensuring that:

1   The names of students, apprentices and learners are understood, remembered, pronounced and spelt correctly?
2   How might you develop your role and practice encompass allyship?
3   What if any aspects of your use of language needs to be developed to ensure that you become the inclusive educator that you want to become?

Conclusion

In this chapter, we have seen that the health and wellbeing of students and apprentices has not only been impacted by the COVID-19 pandemic, but is inextricably linked to their lived experience within all practice education experiences, which may be deep and profound. The needs of the failing student and the student in difficulty require practice supervisors, assessors and educators to undertake a comprehensive and holistic assessment that differentiates between the identification of causes of concern, student welfare and fitness to practice. Enabling students, apprentices and other supervisors to adopt a developmental approach to action planning is critical to protecting the best interests of learners, enables students and apprentices to succeed and provides evidence to support assessment decision-making. Finally, we saw that the provision of inclusive as well as compassionate practice learning environments is of strategic importance to the challenging of injustice, oppression and discriminatory practice, which operate in hidden systemic ways as well as more overtly through the use of language.

References

Ajjawi, R, Dracup, M, Zacharias, N, Bennett, S, Boud, D (2020) 'Persisting students' explanations of and emotional responses to academic failure', *Higher Education Research & Development*, 39 (2), pp. 185–199, 10.1080/07294360.2019.1664999

Askham, P (2008) 'Context and identity: Exploring adult learners' experiences of higher education', *Journal of Further & Higher Education*, 32 (1), pp. 85–97.

Biesta, G, Tedder, M (2016) 'Agency and learning in the life course: Towards an ecological perspective', *Studies in the Education of Adults*, 39 (2), pp. 132–149.

Borrott, N, Day, GE, Sedgwick, M, Levett-Jones, T (2016) Nursing students' belongingness and workplace satisfaction: Quantitative findings of a mixed methods study. *Nurse Education Today*, 45, pp. 29–34.

Couper, K, Murrells, T, Sanders, J, Anderson, JE, Blake, H, Kelly, D, Kent, B, Maben, J, Rafferty, AM, Taylor, RM, Harris, R (2022) 'The impact of COVID-19 on the wellbeing of the UK nursing and midwifery workforce during the first pandemic wave: A longitudinal survey study', *International Journal of Nursing Studies*, 127, p. 104155, 10.1016/j.ijnurstu.2021.104155. Epub 15 December 2021. PMID: 35093740; PMCID: PMC8673915.

CSP (2021) *Common placement assessment form*. London: Chartered Society of Physiotherapists. https://www.csp.org.uk/professional-clinical/practice-based-learning/cpaf

Gillen, T (2008). *Negotiating, Influencing and Persuading Chartered*. London: Institute of Personnel & Development.

Grimsley, A (2010). *Vital Conversations Barnes Holland*. Princes Risborough: Barnes Holland.

Hammond, JA, Williams, A, Walker, A, Norris, M (2019) 'Working hard to belong: A qualitative study exploring students from black, Asian and minority ethnic backgrounds experiences of pre-registration physiotherapy education', *BMC Medical Education*, 19, p. 372, 10.1186/s12909-019-1821-6

Hamshire, C, Willgoss, TG, Wibberley, C (2013) 'Should I stay or should I go? A study exploring why healthcare students consider leaving their programme', *Nurse Education Today*, 33 (8), pp. 889–895, 10.1016/j.nedt.2012.08.013

Health and Safety Executive (2022) *Work-related stress, anxiety or depression statistics in Great Britain, 2022*. Work-related stress, anxiety or depression statistics in Great Britain, 2022 (hse.gov.uk)

Hou, T, Zhang, T, Cai, W, Song, X, Chen, A, Deng, G, Ni, C (2020) 'Social support and mental health among health care workers during Coronavirus Disease 2019 outbreak: A moderated mediation model'. *PLoS ONE*, 15 (5), p. e0233831.

King-Okoye, M, Arber, A (2014) 'It stays with me': the experiences of second- and third-year student nurses when caring for patients with cancer. *European Journal of Cancer Care*, 23 (4), 441–449.

Lamb, D et al. (2022) 'Capturing the experiences of UK healthcare workers during the COVID-19 pandemic: A structural topic modelling analysis of 7,412 free-text survey responses', *PLoS ONE*, 17 (10), pp. 1–21, 10.1371/journal.pone.0275720

Levett-Jones, T, Lathlean, J, Higgins, I, & McMillan, M (2009a) Staff-student relationships and their impact on nursing students' belongingness and learning. *Journal of Advanced Nursing*, 65 (2), pp. 316–324.

Levett-Jones , T, Lathlean , J (2009b) The ascent to competence conceptual framework: an outcome of a study of belongingness. *Journal of Clinical Nursing*, 18 (20), pp. 2870–2879.

Mandy, A, Tucker, B, Tinley, P (2006) 'Sources of stress in undergraduate podiatry students in the UK and Australia … including commentary by Maville JA, Dahlin M, Dutta A', *International Journal of Therapy & Rehabilitation*, 13 (3), pp. 109–117, 10.12968/ijtr.2006. 13.3.21362

McFadden, P, Neill, RD, Mallett, J, Manthorpe, J, Gillen, P, Moriarty, J, Currie, D, Schroder, H, Ravalier, J, Nicholl, P, Ross, J (2022) 'Mental well-being and quality of working life in UK social workers before and during the COVID-19 pandemic: A propensity score matching study', *British Journal of Social Work*, 52 (5), pp. 2814–2833, 10.1093/bjsw/bcab198

Mercer, J (2007) 'Re-negotiating the self through educational development: Mature students' experiences', *Research in Post-Compulsory Education*, 12 (1), pp. 19–32.

Najimi, A, Shafirad, G, Amini, MM, Meftagh, SD (2013) 'Academic failure and students' viewpoint: The influence of individual, internal and external organizational factors', *Journal of Education & Health Promotion*, 2 (22), 10.4103%2F2277-9531.112698

Nixon, SA (2019) 'The coin model of privilege and allyship: implications for health', *BMC Public Health*, 19, p. 1637, 10.1186/s12889-019-7884-9

NMC (2023) Standards for student supervision and assessment, London, Nursing & Midwifery Council. At: https://www.nmc.org.uk/standards-for-education-and-training/standards-for-student-supervision-an d-assessment/

Sedgwick , M, Oosterbroek , T, Ponomar , V (2014). "It all depends": how minority nursing students experience belonging during clinical experiences. *Nursing Education Perspectives*, 35 (2), pp. 89–93.

Wainwright, E, Marandet, E (2010) 'Parents in higher education: Impacts of university learning on the self and the family', *Educational Review*, 62 (4), pp. 449–465.

Wallace, L, Bourke, MP, Tormoehlen, LJ, Poe-Greskamp, MV (2015) Perceptions of Clinical Stress in Baccalaureate Nursing Students. *International Journal of Nursing Education Scholarship*, 12 (1), pp. 91–98.

Wareing, M, Newberry-Baker, R, Sharples, A, Pye, S (2024) Career motivation of 1st year nursing and midwifery students: A cross-sectional study, *International Journal of Practice Learning in Health & Social Care* [forthcoming].

Wojecki, A (2016) "What's identity got to do with it, anyway?' Constructing adult learner identities in the workplace', *Studies in the Education of Adults*, 39 (2), pp. 168–182.

Chapter 8

Compassionate and ethical practice learning

Mark Wareing and Adrienne Sharples

By the end of this chapter you will be able to:

1 Explore the importance of quality in the delivery of compassionate and ethical practice learning.
2 Explain at least four key features of an educational audit.
3 Discuss the role of university link lectures/tutors in the support of practice supervisors, assessors, educators and students/apprentices.
4 Describe the role of a range of key stakeholders in resolving issues arising from a dissatisfied student or apprentice.

Introduction

Compassionate and ethical practice learning environments are reliant on a continuous quality enhancement approach that places the learner experience at the heart of workplace learning. This chapter will explore the key quality enhancement requirements that underpin the work of practice supervisors, assessors and educators and ensure that practice education is delivered in an effective, valid and reliable manner. Increasingly, professional standard regulatory bodies require evidence of robust partnership and collaborative working to enhance learning for all students and apprentices in accordance with regulatory educational standards and assessment requirements. In this chapter, partnership working will be understood as the working relationship between practice partners and approved education institutes, whereas collaborative working is the nature of the co-creative activity or joint development work critical to the provision of compassionate and ethical practice learning environments and resolving where possible, concerns raised by dissatisfied students and apprentices.

Educational auditing

Traditionally, approved education institutes such as universities have played a key role in working with practice partners within all clinical, therapeutic or service settings to complete educational audits of workplace, clinical area, team or therapeutic areas. Whilst audit documents vary between universities, the document template will normally include information such as:

DOI: 10.4324/9781003358602-8

- Name, location, address, telephone numbers of placement; key contacts, including the educational link/nominated person, learning environment lead, head of education training and university link lecturer/tutor;
- Pre-placement reading list, websites, key policies, strategy documents or common procedures, treatment and management pathways;
- Placement capacity including number of students, study pathways and student allocation by academic year;
- Practice learning opportunities, members of the multidisciplinary team that students and apprentices can shadow and work alongside;
- Record of the establishment of practice supervisors, assessors and educators; their training details and names of staff requiring training or updates.

The completion of the audit will also include a substantive piece of work to evaluate the learning environment against a range of criteria (typically mapped against professional standard regulatory body standards) requiring the auditors to identify evidence within the environment sufficient to meet the criteria. In order to demonstrate sufficient confidence relating to the range of evidence, the auditor may 'RAG-rate' each standard on the basis of 'red' (unable to meet the standard), 'amber' (partially meets the standard) or 'green' (fully meets the standard) ratings. Red or amber RAG-rated standards usually require written commentary to justify the RAG-rating outcome and result in an action plan, with each action explicitly referenced to the corresponding standard. Educational auditing is normally completed with a link lecturer/tutor or senior educator from a university, the education link/nominated person for the placement area and a member of the practice partner's practice education team. This tripartite strategy promotes collaboration, which is particularly important in ensuring the actions arising from the audit are owned by all parties and completed within a timely manner. As we saw in Chapter 2, a key feature of educational auditing is an assessment of placement capacity, which, according to Borwell and Leigh (2021), can only be realised when three interdependent conditions are explored:

1 **Function:** the identification of practice learning opportunities that support the learner in meeting their programme's intended learning outcomes, leading to professional registration.
2 **Size of service:** comprising of factors including service hours, the nature of the workforce and workplace environment.
   Borwell and Leigh (2021) suggest that a service that operates full time has greater potential capacity compared to a part-time service. Therefore, whole-time-equivalent (WTE) staff are a useful indicator of size of service, although caution should be exercised by auditors if used in isolation as there maybe a higher proportion of WTE staff in some clinical, therapeutic or specialised areas.
3 **Ability:** arguably, the most significant element, focusing on the need for sufficient supervision and assessment from suitably prepared staff with dedicated time to undertake the roles.

Again, Borwell and Leigh (2021) argue that whatever the function and size of a service, without ability, potential placement capacity will remain unused. Ability is contingent on what can be safely achieved while maintaining quality, person-centred care. Limited capacity is often conflated with limited ability, particularly when a service has a poor skill mix following the employment of new qualified registered professionals or where there has been a high turnover of staff. In such a situation, the impact is on ability, rather than the function or the size of the service.

Activity I

As we have seen, it is commonplace for each clinical or therapeutic area that supports students and apprentices to have had an educational audit completed.

1   Contact your education link or 'nominated person' to locate the most current educational audit for your practice area. This may be stored in the workplace practice placement portfolio.
2   Examine the document and identify:

- When the audit was completed and the expiry date.
- The range of students and apprentices, including professional group, programme/ field, year of study and from which university.
- Whether the reading/resource list would adequately prepare a student to participate in care when undertaking a placement or practice experience within your area.
- The extent to which the audit describes the range of learning opportunities available and whether they cater for the range of students indicated within the placement capacity section.

3   Compare and contrast the current educational audit document with your student/ apprentice welcome pack and identify:

- Whether the welcome pack captures all of the current learning opportunities available for students/apprentices as reflected in the audit.
- The extent to which students/apprentices would be able to arrange to spend time with members of the multidisciplinary team and whether this is indicated in the audit.
- If the audit contains a current risk assessment sufficient to safeguard all students, apprentices and learners and whether this is reflected in guidance and information sufficient to promote the health, safety and well-being of students, within the welcome pack.

A key responsibility of educational links/nominated persons is to ensure that the placement area has an up-to-date student welcome pack that is not only closely aligned but reflects the content of the most recent educational audit. When creating a new placement, it is sometimes useful to ask a student to review and suggest ways in which the welcome pack can be enhanced, with the inclusion of learning opportunities and suggestions for self-directed learning activities and emailed to students prior to their arrival.

Working with universities

In addition to the preparation and maintenance of the learning environment through auditing, practice partners work with universities to directly support students and apprentices and to respond to their learning, wellbeing and assessment needs. As we saw in Chapter 5, the key components of assessment include formative (developmental or 'mid-point) assessments as well as summative, final assessments which are pass or fail. The next activity demonstrates the importance of strong and effective relationships between practice partners and universities, using assessment as an example.

Activity 2

Trixie, a second-year physiotherapy student, failed a summative assessment during her final placement within a cardio-thoracic unit in a large city-based NHS teaching hospital. Prior to her placement, Trixie had experienced a family bereavement and took a small amount of sick leave due to an acute illness. Unfortunately, due to staff sickness, her mid-point assessment was not completed and her allocated practice educator changed twice, whilst the clinical area had been supporting apprentices and direct entry students from four different regional universities. Naturally, Trixie was deeply upset to have failed her practice assessment, which she perceived was due to circumstances beyond her control and felt the assessment outcome was unexpected. Having spoken to her parents, Trixie sought impartial advice from the university student support services.

1 What, if any, mitigating factors may have contributed to the outcome of Trixie's summative assessment?
2 What form of evidence will be required in order for Trixie to substantiate her claim regarding her circumstances?
3 What advice might the university student support service provide?
4 Who would be able to support Trixie throughout this difficult time?

Hopefully, the above vignette will have reminded you of topics such as practice assessment and action planning covered in Chapter 5 as well as the importance of giving effective feedback in Chapter 6. We will return to the story of Trixie as a prelude to considering the type of support provided by universities in such a situation:
    The university student support service recommended that Trixie lodge an academic appeal against her practice assessment fail, which she submits after the Examination Board takes place, following the completion of her cardiothoracic placement. Additionally, Trixie is advised to seek impartial advice and support from the students' union by her personal academic tutor. Trixie's academic appeal application is independently assessed by an appropriate senior academic within the university, in accordance with the academic appeals process.
    Her appeal is upheld on the grounds that:

• *she did not have sufficient opportunity for a mid-point assessment;*
• *a mid-point assessment may have identified her developmental needs, leading to an action plan;*

- *support from practice educators was disruptive;*
- *there was no documentary evidence within Trixie's practice assessment documentation relating to her developmental needs or the impact of missed clinical hours arising from sickness.*

The university director of practice learning is notified of the outcome of the academic appeal by the physiotherapy programme lead and decides to contact the NHS trust learning environment lead to arrange an appreciative inquiry meeting with Trixie's practice educators and the link lecturer for the cardiothoracic unit. Trixie is informed of both the outcome of the appeal and the response of the university prior to her starting her recovery placement within a different acute area:

1   What might be the emotional reaction of the practice educators when they learn of the outcome of the academic appeal?
2   What outcomes might the following stakeholders be looking for as a result of the appreciative inquiry meeting:

- NHS trust learning environment lead?
- Practice educators?
- Link lecturer?
- Trixie?

It is likely that the practice educators will express dismay at the outcome of the appeal, as they may perceive that their assessment decision has not been valued by the university. Additionally, the practice educators may feel deflation, particularly if they perceive that they did the best they could for Trixie under difficult circumstances, whilst supporting a diverse range of students and may feel anxious at attending a meeting with academic staff from the university.

   The purpose of the appreciative inquiry meeting is for all parties to identify lessons learnt from the support of Trixie and the appeal outcome, although it would not be necessary for her to attend unless she expressed a desire to do so. The NHS trust learning environment lead is a key stakeholder as they have a responsibility to ensure that the cardiothoracic unit is able to support the current capacity of students based on the current staff establishment and availability of practice educators. Trixie's practice educators are key stakeholders as they have a responsibility to be accountable for their assessment decisions, which must follow the assessment strategy and requirements within the practice assessment documentation. The link lecturer will want to attend the meeting to represent the university, support and reassure the practice educators that their assessment decision is valued, to answer any questions regarding the appeals process and seek assurance regarding assessment practice as it affects current students within the unit. Whilst Trixie may or may not want to attend the meeting, it is important that she is informed of the nature and outcome of the meeting, so that she can be assured that fellow or future students will be assessed in a fair, open and transparent manner. Additionally, Trixie may wish to submit a complaint regarding the incident, in accordance with the trust's complaints policy, but would normally be advised to seek a form of mediation prior to embarking on a formal process, which could be stressful and lengthy.

Understanding and responding to complaints and concerns

Practice partners, university practice education and academic staff may receive a range of complaints and concerns from dissatisfied students and apprentices that may be lodged formally, through the submission of a written complaint, or informally, perhaps arising from an opportunistic conversation held with an educator at a student forum meeting or following a taught session at university. Additionally, complaints and concerns may also be shared with university placement administrative staff or be identified from end-of-placement student feedback surveys.

Complaints or concerns normally relate to the following areas:

1   **The quality of the learning environment**: practice supervisor, assessor and educator support and relationships, completion of practice documentation and scheduling of meetings and range of learning opportunities and perceived value of the placement or learning experience.
2   **The quality of the working environment**: staff to student/apprentice ratio; super-nummery status; workload, clinical/patient acuity or throughput; staff skill mix and resources; levels of workplace stress including patient/client service user aggression, abuse or hostility; quality of working relationships between staff and effectiveness of management and leadership within the immediate team, department or ward.
3   **Patient/client service user safety, safeguarding concerns**: near misses, ineffective or poor communicative actions (verbal, non-verbal, documentary); unsafe, inept, illegal practices and fraud; medication management errors; poor adherence or disregard towards policies, standard operating procedures and local and national guidelines; vulnerable adult, children and young people; elderly/frail elderly safeguarding issues; health and safety concerns/incidents/accidents; poor or lack of raising concerns; lack/absence of a learning culture or emphasis on lessons learnt and significant or high level of patient/client/service user complaints and dissatisfaction.

In addition to the above, students and apprentices may make a complaint or raise a concern that may feature a constellation of issues that will require careful contextualisation and timely escalation to key decision-makers at the university and to the practice partner. In the case of a patient safety or safeguarding concern, practice supervisors and assessors should act without delay if they believe that there is a risk to patient safety or public protection (NMC, 2019). Similarly, HCPC-registered practice educators must report any concerns about the safety or well-being of service users promptly and appropriately (HCPC, 2019). A key concept that students and apprentices need to understand in the context of raising a concern is the professional duty of candour, which requires all health and social care professionals to be open and transparent when things go wrong. Joint guidance from the General Medical, Nursing and Midwifery Councils (2022b) states that health and care professionals must:

- tell the person (or, where appropriate, their advocate, carer or family) when something has gone wrong;
- apologise to the person (or, where appropriate, their advocate, carer or family);
- offer an appropriate remedy or support to put matters right (if possible);

- explain fully to the person (or, where appropriate, their advocate, carer or family) the short- and long-term effects of what has happened.

Additionally, health and care professionals must also be open and honest with their colleagues, employers and relevant organisations (such as universities) and take part in reviews and investigations when requested (GMC/NMC, 2022a).

Activity 3

In Chapter 2, you were asked to undertake an exercise to identify and reflect on your personally held values and beliefs.

With reference to the duty of candour requirements in the above section:

1   Identify the professional values and beliefs that you hold dear.
2   To what extent are your professional values and beliefs congruent (in agreement) or incongruent (not in agreement or harmony) with the GMC/NMC (2022a) duty of candour standards?
3   How would you respond if a student or apprentice told you that they could not raise a concern or admit to a patient, client or service user when something went wrong because they thought it was disloyal or they could lose their job?

Universities within the United Kingdom are committed to widening participation in higher education and are required to submit statistics relating to the social and economic backgrounds of their students to the government who produce annual reports available on the GOV.UK website. As a consequence, students/apprentices may come from communities where there may be historic mistrust of local authorities or law enforcement officers, which may mean that they struggle with the requirement to raise a concern and the duty of candour. Practice supervisors, assessors and educators need to exercise sensitivity and a non-judgemental attitude whilst signposting students and apprentices to employer policies and publications from professional regulatory standard bodies that outline the process and sources of support for all health and social care professionals.

Students raising concerns

A systematic literature review into students raising concerns in practice undertaken by Milligan et al. (2017) concluded that barriers to reporting include a lack of clarity with regard to definition of the concepts 'raising concerns' and 'whistle-blowing' and that students perceive that raising concerns might adversely affect their assessment outcomes and progress within placements. Students bring a fresh pair of eyes to practice environments that can allow them to see, sometimes more clearly than permanent staff, the limitations and strengths of the care and treatment being delivered. However, Milligan et al. (2017) noted that students may not always evaluate the quality of care accurately, perhaps due to a lack of knowledge and experience, but as transitory members of staff they will bring a different and potentially useful perspective. Consequently, students and apprentices should be encouraged to consider the nature and process of decision-making when considering raising and escalating a particular concern.

The 'what, when, why, whom' decision-making tool

The tool in Figure 7.1 enables learners to consider the key features of a patient, client or service user incident and provides a step-by-step process for decision-making that can be used to complement practice partner policies and guidance provided by professional standard regulatory bodies (NMC, 2019) (Figure 8.1).

Universities normally advise students/apprentices to submit a written statement of untoward incidents, near misses or patient/client safety concerns, with the support of a personal academic tutor to write a factual, objective, value-free, contemporaneous account featuring the actual words spoken by all people involved who should be clearly identified in terms of their names and job titles (RCN, 2023). There is an expectation that complaints made by students relating to the quality of the working and learning environment are managed initially on an informal basis, in accordance with the practice partner's and university complaints policies. However, students and apprentices have a right to pursue a formal complaint and should be directed to impartial sources of support, should they wish to do so, such as the university student support services, students' union, trade union or the practice partner's freedom to speak up champion or professional advocate.

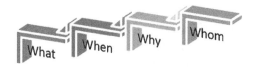

WHAT...	WHEN...	WHY...	WHOM...
have you seen?	will you reflect on what you have seen?	did the incident occur?	will you contact to help you make sense of what you have seen?
people have been involved?	will you gather information that will help you make sense of what you have seen?	did you become conscious of your concern?	will need to be made aware that you intend to raise a concern?
was said?			
was done?		did other people, if any, raise their concerns?	
has not been done?	will you access policies on raising a concern?		
are the possible implications of what you have seen?		might other people not raise a concern?	will need to be contacted to help you write a statement?
concerns do you have?	is the right time for you to report your concern?	if ever, did this happen before?	will support you through the entire process?
		has this not happened before?	

Figure 8.1 'What, when, why, whom' decision-making tool.

Learner expectations

Students and apprentices will have a range of expectations relating to their placement and practice education experiences, which can be positively shaped through the provision of a student welcome pack, which should be sent to the learner ahead of the commencement of the scheduled placement. Naturally, students and apprentices will expect to be welcomed to the workplace area and feel that they 'belong'. Levett-Jones and Lathlean (2008) drew attention to the importance of belongingness within clinical placements for nursing students and argued that the level of belongingness had a direct impact on students' motivation to learn and was a prerequisite for clinical learning. Recent research into career aspirations of nursing and midwifery students (Wareing et al., 2024) suggests that students are more likely to endorse intrinsic motivating factors, such as helping and caring for people, providing a useful role for society and gaining intellectual stimulation over extrinsic factors such as pay, qualifications and career stability when choosing their career. The identification of the motivational factors of students and apprentices provides practice supervisors, assessors and educator with important information that can assist in the management of student expectations, particularly when commencing a new placement or practice experience. Asking students/apprentices what motivated them to choose their career or apprenticeship when starting a new placement, or what motivations they have to place learning at the centre of care might be useful when seeking to identify and enhance students' motivation. Newberry-Baker et al.'s (2023) study demonstrated that previous care employment is a significant factor in the experience of belongingness on placements. Students who had informal care experience reported lower levels of belonging than those with no healthcare experience or with formal employment experience. Therefore, investment on the part of the practice supervisor, assessor or educator to get to know the student/apprentice will assist in the socialisation of learner and recognises that placement and practice education experiences have a significant impact on the emotional wellbeing and career direction of the learner.

Working with link lecturers/tutors

In this activity, we will consider an example of how the role of university link lecturers/ tutors can support students and apprentices to manage difficult situations such as incivility, which can negatively impact their sense of belonging within the practice environment.

Activity 4

Michaela is a lecturer in children's and young people's nursing and link lecturer for the children's unit and paediatric accident and emergency department within an acute NHS hospital in the same city as the university. Every four to six weeks she visits her allocated areas to meet with practice staff and any students on duty. One afternoon, she encounters Desai, a second-year apprentice nursing associate, who is sat alone in the staff room and appears tearful and withdrawn. Michaela has never met Desai before, but learns that they have experienced incivility from a member of staff that is perceived as being racially motivated. Evidently, Desai had been struggling with a drug calculation during a drug round, when the practice supervisor became impatient and spoke to another member of staff in their native language using a phrase that Desai was able to recognise and associated with Desai's tribal heritage.

Imagine that you were Desai's allocated practice supervisor and receive a phone call from Michaela:

1   What actions would you take during the phone call?
2   On what basis would you escalate your concerns and to whom?
3   What are Desai's practice learning needs and how can they be addressed?
4   What key documents or strategies within the NHS trust could be used as a basis for challenging incivility and barriers to civility?

Although Michaela has not met Desai before, as a representative of the university she has quite rightly engaged with a student who is studying a different programme; not least, as Desai is on placement within one of Michaela's placement areas. It is likely that Michaela will not only escalate her concerns regarding Desai to the nursing associate academic team, but provide a summary report of her visits and actions which will be shared with other link lecturers associated with the clinical area and used as evidence of partnership working by the university. The above vignette is a reminder that link lecturers visit placement areas not necessarily to meet students and their practice supervisors, assessors or educators. Michaela identified when Desai's allocated supervisor is next on duty so that she can escalate her concerns directly. This is an important first step in supporting the student and seeking to escalate, albeit informally, a concern expressed by a student who may not necessarily be comfortable with the matter being reported to the ward manager. Clearly, such an incident threatens the wellbeing of Desai. Her sense of belongingness within the ward has been threatened by a possible racial slur, which would need careful investigation should a formal complaint be lodged by Desai. Michaela may cite the NHS trust's statement of organisational values to place in context her concerns regarding Desai's welfare and the shared expectations of all of the practice partner's employees. An NHS acute hospital or community NHS trust values are normally found on the organisation's website. A cursory internet search using the search term *'Our Trust values'* is a useful way of discovering the organisational commitment statements that characterise contemporary health and social care service provision within the United Kingdom.

Universities and practice partners often collect end-of-placement feedback using surveys and questionnaires that are typically completed by students/apprentices online or opportunistically via smartphone QR codes located within the practice area. The 'learner experience' is often regarded as pivotal to the monitoring of the quality of the learning environment, as we shall see in the next activity.

Activity 5

Toby, the trust learning environment lead, arranges an online drop-in session for all education links/nominated persons within the community NHS trust, which is attended by 25 colleagues, all allied health professionals supporting practice educators in a range of clinical, therapeutic and community teams within a large rural area. At the end of the meeting, Toby explains that one of the universities is now collecting quarterly end-of-placement feedback using a digital platform that also hosts the practice assessment documentation. Given the range of placement areas, the feedback will be shared on an 'exception reporting' basis, where particularly positive or less-than-positive feedback is shared with Toby, who in turns escalates reports to individual placement areas. A week after the drop-in session, you receive an email that contains a report of feedback from students who have completed placements within your team over the previous four months. The report contains the following:

85% of students were either 'satisfied' or 'very satisfied' with the student welcome pack
55% of students reported not having an allocated practice educator by the end of the first working week

The following free-text comments were also shared in the report:

'My practice educator could not pronounce my first name and decided to shorten it ... '
"One of my practice educators asked me if there were many male students on my programme and then said she felt that male therapists were only interested in managerial roles'
'There was a client who clearly identified themselves as non-binary during an initial assessment. One of the rehabilitation support workers challenged the therapist when they described the client using a binary gender pronoun, but the therapist ignored the challenge and proceeded to document the assessment using the pronoun'

Toby, the learning environment lead, arranges a meeting with you and your team leader to discuss the most recent feedback, as he will be expected to feedback at the next quarterly quality enhancement meeting where all the universities meet to discuss practice learning within the trust. As education link/nominated person how might you:

1   Ensure that you are supported at the meeting?
2   Interrogate the findings of the report?
3   Contextualise the findings with reference to other sources of feedback relating to the learner experience?
4   Use the feedback to support the team leader to restore a more inclusive and compassionate learning environment?

As an education link/nominated person for your department, ward or team, it would be advisable to ensure that the head of department, line manager or team lead not only has sight of the feedback report but can be present at the meeting, not least as the implications of the feedback suggest issues relating to incivility and discriminatory practices. The report would need to be interrogated in terms of:

1   Whether the feedback has been provided by the participants anonymously.
2   The relationship between the feedback and the allocation of the students; in particular, feedback that relates to a period of challenge or difficulty for the team

and the specific timeline associated with challenging service delivery periods, patient/client acuity and the student allocation.

3   The size of the sample of feedback against the actual number of students allocated during the corresponding placement allocation period.

4   Evidence of patient safety or safeguarding concerns.

Additionally, the learning environment lead could be asked to provide earlier sets of student feedback that could be used for the purposes of triangulation, which would enable a more nuanced critical evaluation and contextualisation of the most recent student feedback. Hopefully, the learning environment lead and departmental lead or manager will want to work collaboratively with the link lecturer/tutor to formulate an action plan to address the particular issues, such as the free-text comments, that point to incivility and a lack of inclusivity.

Conclusion

In this chapter, we explored educational auditing as an essential element of the quality enhancement of placements and its relationship to placement capacity, learning opportunities and the creation of student welcome packs. Auditing provides practice partners with an opportunity to formally review each placement experience to ensure that students and apprentices are provided with expansive learning environments for the benefit of all practitioners and trainees. We saw that the role of link lecturers/tutors is particularly important in supporting students and apprentices undertaking practice-based assessment and that regular visits to clinical and service areas afford university staff with opportunities to identify issues and to provide early intervention. Link lecturers/tutors have a key role in supporting practice assessors, supervisors and educators to undertake open, fair and transparent assessments and be involved in appreciative inquiry when things go wrong. The dissatisfaction of students and apprentices is often associated with the quality of the learning, working and clinical environment, including patient safety or safeguarding concerns or incidents that are a constellation of issues and concerns. A key responsibility of practice supervisors, assessors and educators is to understand the relationship between professional and personally held beliefs and values, raising concerns and the duty of candour. Lastly, we saw that effective collaborative working is necessary when managing student/apprentice expectations, exploring experiences such as incivility and sustaining a compassionate learning environment.

References

Borwell, J, Leigh, J (2021) 'Addressing the practice learning and placement capacity conundrum', *British Journal of Nursing*, 30 (918), p. 1093.

GMC/NMC (2022a) *Openness and honesty when things go wrong: The professional duty of candour*. London: General Medical Council/Nursing & Midwifery Council. https://www.nmc.org.uk/globalassets/sitedocuments/nmc-publications/openness-and-honesty-professional-duty-of-candour.pdf

GMC/NMC (2022b). Guidance on the professional duty of candour, London, General Medical Council and Nursing, Midwifery Council. At: https://www.nmc.org.uk/standards/guidance/the-professional-duty-of-candour/

HCPC (2019) *Standards of conduct, performance and ethics*. London: Health and Care Professions Council. https://www.hcpc-uk.org/globalassets/resources/standards/standards-of-conduct-performance-and-ethics.pdf

Levett-Jones, T, Lathlean, J (2008) 'Belongingness: A prerequisite for nursing students' clinical learning', *Nurse Education in Practice*, 8 (2), pp. 103–111, 10.1016/j.nepr.2007.04.003. Epub 31 May 2007.

Milligan, F, Wareing, M, Preston-Shoot, M, Pappas, Y, Randhawa (2017) 'Supporting nursing, midwifery and allied health professional students to raise concerns with the quality of care: A review of the research literature', *Nurse Education Today*, 57, pp. 29–39, https://www.sciencedirect.com/science/article/abs/pii/S0260691717301466

NMC (2019) *Raising concerns: Guidance for nurses, midwives and nursing associates*. London: Nursing & Midwifery Council. https://www.nmc.org.uk/globalassets/blocks/media-block/raising-concerns-v2.pdf

RCN (2023) *Statements: How to write them*. London: Royal College of Nursing. https://www.rcn.org.uk/Get-Help/RCN-advice/statements#:~:text=Keep%20patients'%20and%20relatives'%20identities,local%20policies%20and%20confidentiality%20guidelines

Wareing, M, Newberry-Baker, R, Sharples, A, Pye, S (2024) Career motivation of 1st year nursing and midwifery students: A cross-sectional study. *International Journal of Practice Learning in Health & Social Care* [forthcoming].

Chapter 9

Practice education in social work

Gillian Ferguson and Sherwyn Sicat

By the end of this chapter, you will be able to:

1 Explain the U.K. context of social work practice education.
2 Discuss the diversity of social work roles, settings and services.
3 Understand the nature of social workers' learning and process of assessment.
4 Describe how to maximise learning in changing workplace contexts including interprofessional/multi-disciplinary settings.

Introduction

In this chapter, we will explore the context of practice education in social work across the United Kingdom (U.K.). We will consider the diverse roles, services and settings in which practitioners work. We will then focus specifically on social work professional practice learning in this landscape. The chapter will consider the nature of social workers' practice learning and assessment in qualifying training and continuing development across career stages. The changing nature of the workplace is considered alongside the needs of these learners. We will consider how to respond to agile working environments and how to maximise learning in multi-disciplinary settings. The chapter provides an overview of practice education for social work for those who are unfamiliar with this and consolidates key information for those who are experienced in this area. It highlights challenges and opportunities and the importance of effective partnership approaches at the individual, organisational and strategic levels for social work practice learning.

Activity 1

Think about social work from your experience and/or knowledge:

- Identify any social work roles, tasks or services that you are familiar with.
- Where does social work take place?
- What do you think are the differences between social work and other health or social care roles? How might this influence learning for social workers?
- What do you know about practice education in social work across the United Kingdom?

DOI: 10.4324/9781003358602-9

If you are experienced in working with social workers or in social work settings, you might have identified several different roles, tasks or where social work takes place. You might be an experienced practice educator or workplace supervisor for social work students or have supported social workers with their continuing learning across their careers. You might have taken a formal or informal role in supporting these learners or be involved in the arrangements for practice placements. Many people will have some knowledge of social work services from work or life experiences, but it can be hard to understand the breadth and scope of these. In the next sections, we will explore the context of social work practice learning across the United Kingdom, the requirements of professional training and the ways in which learning is facilitated and assessed.

Social work service provision

Social workers are often, but not always, practising in social care services and settings, but it is important not to conflate the roles, tasks or protected title with social care. Often social care practice will dovetail with social work, but there is a risk in diluting and misrepresenting each of these if they are seen as a homogenous workforce. Social work has a broad and visionary international definition that is prominent in rhetoric:

> *Social work is a practice-based profession and an academic discipline that promotes social change and development, social cohesion, and the empowerment and liberation of people. Principles of social justice, human rights, collective responsibility and respect for diversities are central to social work. Underpinned by theories of social work, social sciences, humanities and indigenous knowledge, social work engages people and structures to address life challenges and enhance wellbeing.*
>
> (International Federation of Social Workers, 2014)

Although this definition is a common point of reference, the actual roles and tasks of social work are notoriously hard to articulate (Moriarty *et al.*, 2015) and renowned for their complexity (Hood, 2018). Social work is described as perpetually at the crossroads (McCulloch and Taylor, 2018). This means that learning to be a social worker and facilitating or assessing that learning are also complex processes (Ferguson, 2022). Understanding the diversity of where social work happens is important in terms of the types of services but also the nature of these unique workplace learning environments (Ferguson, 2023).

Unlike many other countries around the world, much of the social work delivered in the United Kingdom is done via statutory services, where it is mandated by legislation to deliver services to the public on behalf of the government. This means that political trends can be argued as one of the most significant influences on social policy, associated expectations and resourcing of social work. There is a requirement that social work practice learning equips students for working in this context, and to undertake statutory tasks primarily associated with assessment and decision-making in care and protection, justice or mental health practice. There are differences in what is understood by statutory settings and the specific requirements across U.K. nations. For example, that one substantive period of practice learning takes place in a statutory setting (SWE, 2023). This does not extend across all U.K. nations, but all are concerned with developing students' capacity to understand and undertake statutory tasks. Although there are variances in wording across nations, essentially accountability for far-reaching significance of decisions being made rests with registered social workers in the United Kingdom (Scottish Government, 2010).

The issue of statutory setting is not as simple as it sounds. Demand for social work placements is high and the supply of placements are subject to very different arrangements across United Kingdom. Chapter 16 of this book outlines the diversity of third-sector social care settings. Third-sector services are also regularly commissioned to provide services that are related to local authority responsibilities thereby blurring what counts as statutory. Within these diverse settings, many different professionals undertake their practice learning, particularly with the dominance of integrated partnerships and multi-disciplinary arrangements, which we explore later in this chapter. Within this partnership context, it is essential to understand the nuances of each profession for learning to be effective.

Journeys into social work

Social work students come from a variety of backgrounds and the inspiration for them joining the profession often comes from connecting with and wishing to embody social work values such as social justice as well as having experience social work intervention themselves or knowing someone who has received an intervention (SWE, 2023). In England, the average age of social worker learners for undergraduate level is 27 years old and for postgraduate was 31 years old (Skills for Care, 2023), but there are variable patterns of recruitment and retention across different nations and regions in the United Kingdom. Age and motivation combined with students also having had experiences that are related to social care, whether that was through paid employment or voluntary work results in a highly diverse and individual student group that brings a wealth of knowledge to their placement. There is a strong focus in social work, as in many other helping professions, in recruiting a workforce that mirrors the demographic patterns of communities so that people who receive services can see people like them. This has been a focus of the anti-racist social work agenda (Reid, 2020) and the movement for inclusion of people who are care-experienced (Carter and Maclean, 2022). Social workers have a parallel trajectory in their personal and professional lives in relation to the impact of learning in practice settings (Ferguson, 2023). This journey for social workers involves connecting with their values, sense of fit with the profession, recognition of the seriousness of the task and development of identity (Ferguson, 2021).

Activity 2

- Are you aware of the differences in social work between areas of the United Kingdom?
- What do you think is important for those supporting social workers' learning to know?
- If you are involved in supporting social workers' learning, do you know where the regulations and guidance are for your geographic or specialist area?

You may not have any direct involvement in social work education or practice learning for this profession. You might support other professionals to learn in social work or social care settings. In contrast, you may be heavily involved as a practice educator or workplace supervisor of social work students or have a leadership role in supporting learning. Most people who are involved have knowledge of their own country, the regulations, guidance and any partnership arrangements within their local areas that support placements. Often, people are surprised at the differences across the United Kingdom, but the essence of practice learning in social work shares more similarities than differences, which we will explore in the next sections. One of the things that is important to know about is what it is like for social workers learning in practice, and how they learn in such diverse settings, to which we now turn.

Understanding how social workers learn in practice

To develop effective learning opportunities for social workers, it is essential to understand what this involves.

> Social work learning is usually understood to include the development of skills and competences which enable practitioners to undertake a role which is rooted in human rights and social justice, where ethical practice needs to be negotiated within a work role where there are competing moral, legal, organisational and policy demands.
>
> (Ferguson, 2021, p. 20)

Figure 9.1 shows *what* social workers learn at the intersection of expectations of their learning learn, how that learning is supported and facilitated but also importantly, how they learn.

In relation to how social workers learn, Ferguson outlines that 'this is a complex, individual, intricate web of physical and emotional elements while learners are navigating places, spaces and tasks' (Ferguson, 2023, p. 2), as shown in Figure 9.2. The different elements of the diagram are linked by multiple threads and connections in relation to the experience of social workers' learning in workplace settings.

We have already thought briefly about the personal journey of a learner in social work, which can involve the creation of a new persona or the integration of different parts of an individual (Ferguson, 2021). The individual social worker finds themselves in practice settings where they are navigating diverse landscapes (Ferguson, 2021).

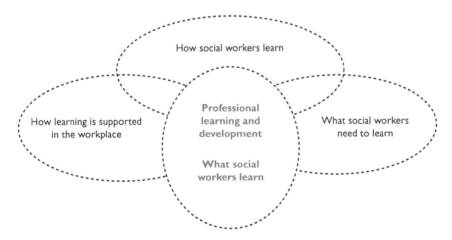

Figure 9.1 Influences on professional learning in the workplace (Ferguson, 2022).

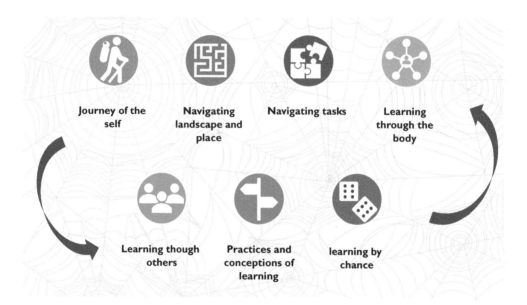

Figure 9.2 Learning in the workplace as a complex web (Ferguson, 2021, p. 154).

We have explored learning environments more broadly in Chapters 1 and 3. For social work, these places are very diverse, such as in a court, hospital ward or domestic setting, and are often physically or psychologically isolated without any overall route map or guidebook. Social work practice when undertaking a home visit is complex, as professional boundaries may be pushed, challenging confident and experienced practitioners (Ferguson, 2009). Navigating social work practice settings also involves the physical, sensory elements of these places. Organisational culture and the physical location of social workers is also an important factor in how learning can be facilitated.

We have outlined the complexity and diversity of social work tasks earlier in the chapter, but this is essential to understand as part of the complex web. In order to plan and support social workers to learn, it is important to consider the types of tasks and multiple sub-tasks within any work allocated. Navigating this complexity is learned through experiential practice, highlighting that direct practice is a primary vehicle for professional learning (Ferguson, 2022). It is impossible to reduce social work to simplistic task definitions or numbers of cases as a measure in allocation yet attempts to do so prevail. As is the case with many health and social care roles, social workers learn in practice about life and death – sometimes literal and other times about important aspects of life and death. Social work is described as an extraordinary job (Ferguson, 2022) where extreme tasks become the ordinary daily work yet remain extraordinary.

Learning through the body is a central element of social workers' learning, including both physical and emotional experience (Ferguson, 2023). Tuning into the details of sensory experiences of the workplace and practice enhances understanding of what is going on for social workers when they are learning. Social work is commonly associated with emotions in practice, but this is rarely defined as emotional labour

(Hochschild, 1983) and less so physical labour, yet this is a central aspect (Ferguson, 2021). The influence of other people on social workers' learning is significant and perhaps not a surprise. The changing nature of organisations in terms of agile working and interprofessional settings means that social workers are not always physically located with one another. Research shows other social workers were critical to social workers' learning through and in workplaces (Ferguson, 2021). Places and spaces for social workers to learn as a single profession have decreased. As the landscape and place of social work continues to change, it is important to ask where the social workers are in your organisation. Learning through direct work with people using the services remains one of the most important elements in any profession and the specific detailed learning that happens through work with individual people is invaluable. Social workers learn in this way throughout their careers, but their initial training embeds a significant direct practice learning component which we will now explore.

Practice education in social work and social care in the United Kingdom

Across the United Kingdom, there is a broad spectrum of social care and social work services for children, young people and adults spanning generic and specialist functions of support and protection across the lifespan. There are different vocational qualifications and degree pathways for social care and qualifying training routes for social workers. There are also different regulatory frameworks for the registration of social workers, social care workers and the regulation of their education, training and continuing professional development (CPD). The regulation of social work and social care in the United Kingdom is an evolving landscape that has developed since 2000, establishing regulatory bodies. At the time of writing, the regulatory function, in terms of social work, is undertaken by Social Work England, Social Care Wales, Northern Ireland Social Care Council and the Scottish Social Services Council, respectively, but arrangements can and do change. The functions of the regulators are concerned with the standards for education and training but also extend to the registration of social workers, their associated fitness to practice and perceived suitability for the profession. The Subject Benchmark Statement for Social Work (QAA, 2019) provides the basis for the knowledge and skills that must be integrated in a social work programme. Formal practice learning requirements are an integral mandatory requirement for all social work programmes in the United Kingdom, with some specific differences in the detailed requirements. Although there are strong similarities in the fundamental principles and essence of U.K. approaches, there are differences in how the regulatory frameworks and practice contexts influence the nuances of practice learning.

Social workers are supported and assessed by a practice educator (PE) who will have undertaken training or qualifications for the role. There are different training programmes and requirements for this across the United Kingdom, but they share a philosophy of ethical assessment and professional focus. Where a PE is not available in the placement setting, a workplace supervisor may be identified and a working alliance developed between the student, an offsite PE and workplace supervisor to support the learning. In any profession and setting, careful negotiation of the boundaries, roles and expectations of practice learning is essential, and care taken at the early stage is valuable should any issues arise. There are different configurations of how the required number of practice learning days are woven into university programmes. There are some slight differences in the numbers of practice learning days required across U.K. nations, and what can count in terms of these.

These issues remain the subject of debate and continuing focus for the profession and those regulating it.

Regulatory standards and guidance on practice learning in social work education include the following:

- The number of days required in assessed practice learning
- The number of days that can be integrated skills days woven into curriculum
- Who can act as a practice educator/assessor and their required qualifications
- Roles, responsibilities and requirements for workplace supervisors
- Expectations relating to practice settings including statutory experience and expected contrast between placements during training
- Potential conflicts of interest and the management of these
- Undertaking placements in own workplace setting if undertaking a work-based programme
- Professional supervision of students in practice

This list is not exhaustive and formal standards are accompanied by detailed guidance. Although there are differences noted in programmes, there are shared core components of social work practice learning in the United Kingdom in terms of the ethos and approach. This includes the centrality of professional supervision in guiding learning, shaping professional identity and modelling a critically reflective space that should continue throughout the social workers' career. Other core elements are the focus on the social worker's use of self (Gordon and Dunworth, 2017) and development of emotional intelligence (Ingram, 2013). Reflective practice is at the heart of practice learning, with students expected to demonstrate their application of theory and legislation to the work they are undertaking. Although the wording and details vary, U.K. standards emphasise the social work role in promoting wellbeing, support and the protection of children and adults across the life span. Assessment and management of risks are also explicit within the role and expectations of competence to be demonstrated. We have explored earlier that social workers learn from one another, but they also undertake practice learning in interprofessional and multi-disciplinary settings, which we will now consider.

Supporting and facilitating learning in interprofessional/multidisciplinary settings

The role of a social worker is unique, and they frequently interact with other professionals and disciplines. Not only do social workers negotiate and advocate for the support of people they are supporting through other services, but they also often work closely with, support and coordinate other professionals to ensure an effective intervention (NCS, 2023). This part of the role is no different for social work students; therefore, understanding the different roles in your team can support you in understanding the various learning opportunities available.

Social work is no longer a role undertaken in isolation but rather one working in partnership with others. This has become embedded in both policy and legislation across the United Kingdom in relation to work with children and adults. In England, for example, SCIE (2009) saw social workers as having more than just formalised links; for example, such as through legislation but rather an active process of collaboration. Social work has gained lessons learned publicly through child deaths (NSPCC, 2018) and adults in homicide reviews (Home Office, 2023). The subject of how students are prepared for interprofessional practice is less studied (Flynn, 2019) compared to a significant body of work related to post-qualifying professional development (Barr, 2011).

Social workers are increasingly found in multi-disciplinary teams such as hospitals, youth offending, community mental health, etc. Settings are multi-disciplinary in that there are a variety of different professionals located within one establishment. They can be seen as interprofessional in that each discipline brings their own perspective in the collaboration process. Barr et al. (2016) argue that there is a compelling case for every student to have at least one placement in an interprofessional team.

Activity 3

Think about a multi-disciplinary setting that you work in or are familiar with. Consider a few of the different professional roles and what learning opportunities are associated with these. For example, this might involve learning more about another person's role or how this supports/enhances a social worker's role.

Look at Table 9.1 and make some notes in the empty boxes. You will note that the first column has been completed as an example.

It is appreciated that the position of a social worker opens opportunities for learning. It also should be appreciated that there are intricacies within the various relationships of a multi-disciplinary team and how these roles can imbue power, position and privilege. For example, in a hospital team, the doctors may be seen as having a greater position of power than a social worker and this may be reinforced in the setting due to their adherence to a medical model of care and the culture of the organisation. As a result, those in more powerful positions may offer a much more limited availability of learning opportunities compared to others. Social workers are often perceived as having power in their roles however often this is a perception rather than actual power. Social workers may have a greater influence in creating opportunities rather than these being offered to them as explored earlier in the chapter due to the diversity of social care settings. This is important when thinking about safeguarding roles where people with accessing services feel obliged to engage or agree in the social care process. Think about who has the most power within multi-disciplinary teams. An example is that lone social workers in palliative care teams can feel marginalised because they work in medical settings (hospices and hospitals). It is also worth considering whether some people may like their positions and work in a way that reinforces their status.

In the early stages of forming multidisciplinary teams, it can be confusing as each profession attempts to establish their professional identity and remit. The overlap in roles can be confusing and understanding who the lead is could be an issue to address early on. There are other issues to think about, such as whether workers in multi-professional teams share a common language. Social work, health and education all have their own

Table 9.1 The role and practice of professionals with multi-disciplinary teams

Profession/role	Registered nurse			
Remit/Focus	Delivery of nursing care to patients and their families			
Strengths of Role to People with Lived Experience	Provides holistic care and range of healthcare interventions including those with enduring or long-term conditions			
Challenges of Role to People with Lived Experience of Social Work	Role and practice operate within clinical setting, where evidence-based practice predominates rather than social determinants of health			
How Does the Profession Support Social Work?	Provides advocacy for patients and their families			
What Is a Learning Opportunity That You Can Engage in with the Profession?	Understanding of contemporary healthcare provision including management of enduring and long-term conditions			

terminology, which can feel alienating to partners and to people accessing the services. Inclusive, anti-discriminatory and anti-oppressive practice is central to multi-disciplinary working for people with lived experience of social work as well as the other professionals who are collaborating. This means considering difference and diversity in planning and delivery of services and actively challenging power imbalances.

Activity 4

Think about a service that you work in or know well:

1 Can you think of any language or habits that are particular to only one of the professions?
2 Are you aware of who leads this service or team? Are certain team members competing for control?
3 Do some professionals have more status than others? How do you know? Who would have the final say in decisions?
4 How do these issues influence the learning opportunities for different professionals? What is it that people learn about one another's roles?

There are no simple answers to the questions in Activity 4 and your experiences may differ from other people. This reflects the complex partnership arena of health and social services. Returning to the focus of learning, all these issues influence the nature of the learning environment for social workers and other professionals and careful planning can maximise enablers to learning and availability of placements. There are complex and dynamic relationships in practice learning in the employer and university context. Developing and managing relationships to support learning are always an important focus and when things go wrong in social work programmes it is often within the practice element due to the complex variables (Finch, 2015).

Conclusion

This chapter has provided an outline of social work roles, services and settings and identified key issues about the nature of practice learning in this profession. Understanding the specific needs of different professions is essential when planning and supporting learning in practice settings. We have considered the context of practice learning for social work within the United Kingdom and explored some of the similarities and differences, noting that there is a shared ethos and approach at the heart. Professional supervision, reflection and learning from people with lived experiences of social work is at the heart of effective learning. Recognising professional learning needs is paramount for effective learning in interprofessional and multi-disciplinary settings, too. Creating an environment that values the unique contributions of everyone to making a difference is the ultimate goal.

References

Barr, H (2011) 'Toward a theoretical framework for interprofessional education', *Journal of Interprofessional Care*, 27(1), pp. 4–9.

Barr, H, Gray, R, Helme, M, Low, H, Reeves, S (2016) *Interprofessional Education Guidelines 2016* [Online], available at https://www.caipe.org/resources/publications/caipe-publications/barr-h-gray-r-helme-m-low-h-reeves-s-2016-interprofessional-education-guidelines (accessed 29 November 2023).

Carter, M, Maclean, S. (eds) (2022) *Insiders outsiders: Hidden narratives of care experienced social workers*. Staffordshire: Kirwin Maclean Associates.

Ferguson, H (2009) 'Performing child protection: Home visiting, movement and the struggle to reach the abused child', *Child and Family Social Work*, 14(4), pp. 471–480.

Ferguson, G (2021) '"When David Bowie created Ziggy Stardust". The lived experiences of social workers learning through work', Milton Keynes, The Open University. Available at http://oro.open.ac.uk/77930/

Ferguson, G (2022) *The importance of workplace learning for social workers*, IRISS, Scotland [Online], available at https://www.iriss.org.uk/resources/insights/importance-workplace-learning-social-workers (accessed 29 November 2023).

Ferguson, G (2023) '"When David Bowie created Ziggy Stardust" Reconceptualising workplace learning for social workers', *The Journal of Practice Teaching and Learning*, 20(1), pp. 67–87.

Finch, J (2015) '"Running with the fox and hunting with the hounds": Social work tutors' experiences of managing failing social work students in practice learning settings', *British Journal of Social Work*, 45 (7), pp. 2124–2141.

Flynn, A (2019) *Preparation of students in education for social work practice in an inter-professional setting*. Unpublished Reference being checked.

Gordon, J, Dunworth, M (2017) 'The fall and rise of "use of self"? An exploration of the positioning of use of self in social work education', *Social Work Education*, 36 (5), pp. 591–603.

Hochschild, AR (1983) *The managed heart: Commercialization of human feeling*. Berkeley: University of California Press.

Home Office (2023) *Domestic homicide review collection* [Online], available at https://www.gov.uk/government/collections/domestic-homicide-review (accessed 10 December 2023).

Hood, R (2018) *Complexity in social work*. London: Sage.

IFSW (2014) Global definition of the docial work profession, International Federation of Social Workers, available at https://www.ifsw.org/what-is-social-work/global-definition-of-social-work/

Ingram, R (2013) 'Locating emotional intelligence at the heart of social work practice', *British Journal of Social Work*, 43 (5), pp. 987–1004.

McCulloch, T, Taylor, S (2018) 'Becoming a social worker: Realising a shared approach to professional learning?', *The British Journal of Social Work*, 48, 2272–2290. 10.1093/bjsw/bcx157

Moriarty, J, Baginsky, M, Manthorpe, J (2015) *Literature review of roles and issues within the social work profession in England*. Social Care Workforce Research Unit, London, King's College London.

National Careers Service (2023) *Social worker* [Online], available at https://nationalcareers.service.gov.uk/job-profiles/social-worker (accessed 29 November 2023).

NSPCC (2018) Case reviews published in 2018 [Online], available at https://www.nspcc.org.uk/preventing-abuse/child-protection-system/case-reviews/2018/ (accessed 16 October 2023).

QAA (2019) Subject benchmark statement social work, Gloucester, Quality Assurance Agency, available at   chrome-extension://efaidnbmnnnibpcajpcglclefindmkaj/https://www.qaa.ac.uk/docs/qaa/subject-benchmark-statements/subject-benchmark-statement-social-work.pdf?%20sfvrsn=5c35c881_6

Reid, W (2020) 'Promoting anti-racism in social work', Research in Practice seminar [Online], available at https://www.researchinpractice.org.uk/all/content-pages/videos/promoting-anti-racism-in-social-work/ (accessed 29 October 2023).

Scottish Government (2010) Role of the registered social worker in statutory interventions: guidance for local authorities, Edinburgh, Scottish Government, available at https://www.gov.scot/publications/role-registered-social-worker-statutory-interventions-guidance-local-authorities/pages/2/

Skills for Care (2023) 'Social work education' [Online], available at https://www.skillsforcare.org.uk/Adult-Social-Care-Workforce-Data/Workforce-intelligence/documents/Social-Work-Education-in-England-2023.pdf (accessed 29 November 2023).

Social Care Institute for Excellence (2009) *Interprofessional and inter-agency collaboration* [Online], available at https://www.communitycare.co.uk/2009/08/03/interprofessional-and-inter-agency-collaboration/ (accessed 29 November 2023).

Social Work England (2023) *Social work in England: State of the nation 2023* [Online], available at https://www.socialworkengland.org.uk/media/4658/social-work-in-england-state-of-the-nation-2023.pdf (accessed 29 November 2023).

Chapter 10

Supporting learners working with children and young people

Tina Salter, Sherwyn Sicat and Mel Webb

By the end of this chapter, you will be able to:

1   Reflect on the nature of children and young people's services, to better understand what supervisory support might be needed in this context.
2   Consider what approaches to learning and development might be most appropriate for students working in children's and young people's services.
3   Draw on family-centred care as a model for supporting students, as they in turn work directly with families.

Contemporary U.K. children and young people service sector

In England, around 2 million young people interact with youth services (National Youth Agency, 2023a). For a number of years, children and youth services have provided much-needed support for young people. Practitioners in this sector have provided early intervention support for young people and their families and it is acknowledged that youth work has a positive impact on children's health and wellbeing, which impacts their academic attainment and attendance (National Youth Agency, 2023b). Despite this contribution, in 2020, 4,500 youth workers had been cut, 760 youth centres closed (YMCA, 2020) and there has been a reduction of 1 billion pounds in spending since 2018/2019 across England and Wales (YMCA, 2023).

The impact of austerity measures has resulted in many youth services adapting in order to continue. Some youth services have been incorporated into the statutory sector while others have been integrated with other services to limit the financial burden of maintaining their own facilities. This multi-agency setting has been reinforced through the support of family hubs (EIF, 2020) and recommendations of the Independent Review of Children's Social Care (MacAlister, 2022).

All these various measures have impacted on supporting learners in children and family services. Closure and cuts have resulted in a limited capacity to provide robust and diverse placements. While the move to multi-disciplinary interventions is a great opportunity for inter-professional learning, the limits in resources could mean less capacity to support and engage learners in an effective and meaningful way.

Prior to the COVID-19 pandemic, the use of remote and hybrid working had been on a steady rise. Upon the arrival of the pandemic, this significantly increased as the country attempted to adapt to an unprecedented situation. This then led to a shift in emphasis from face-to-face worker interactions with children and young people to

DOI: 10.4324/9781003358602-10

engagement with them on digital platforms. For some young people, the pandemic was a reprieve from the everyday stresses of the busyness of school and everyday life. For others, the isolation had an impact on emotional wellbeing and the isolation limited much needed social interaction. Targeted support was identified on how to engage young people during such a significant time. While young people engaging on digital platforms was not new, children and young workers needed more time to adapt their practice. A hybrid engagement of face-to-face and online continues to be offered today and this means of interaction has both benefits and challenges for both young people and their workers.

While placement capacity in health and social care had already been a challenge for several years, the onset of the pandemic intensified this shortage. The limited placement opportunities meant complications for graduates completing their programmes and participating in the workforce. To alleviate this issue, online placements began to be offered, and these opportunities have gradually grown even once pandemic restrictions were lifted.

For a number of professions, simulated placements have become viable options, and an increasing number of simulated hours are being incorporated into study programmes. This then raises questions as to the necessary skills and technological literacy that students need to possess within an online placement and whether they can effectively engage in the process to obtain the necessary skills for online practice in the future. Overall, it raises the question, is it safe and suitable for students to undertake online placements and are they ready to work in the children and young person field?

Other developments are the noted skills shortages in several sectors of the U.K. workforce. Higher technical education, such higher national certificate and higher national diplomas, were seen as possible solution for individuals to unlock these opportunities and obtain well paid jobs. However a limited number were studying via these routes and the introduction of higher technical qualifications introduced in 2023 was seen to address this. These Level 4 and 5 qualifications were seen as an alternative to degrees and apprenticeships, allowing students to complete courses based on virtual placements, removing the need for face-to-face experiences. Whilst this offers flexibility, there are concerns regarding the potential limits of this mode of study for students in training to work directly with people with complex needs.

Implications for placement supervisor's practice

A number of factors have influenced the contemporary U.K. children and young people's service sector, some of which has been outlined above related to more significant aspects over recent years. These factors influence the student's learning environment and can impact what learning opportunities are available. The supervisor needs to carefully consider the students' context and how they can support and hinder the learning environment for the student.

Activity 1

In this first activity, you will be asked to assess the context of the placement how it could impact the learning environment for the student:

1   Which of the above factors could impact your practice environment?

2   Are there other prominent contextual or political situations at the moment that could influence the quality of your placement learning environment? Consider how these might present as benefits and challenges, in relation to learning opportunities for students and apprentices.
3   What support might the student or apprentice need from you as their supervisor, or the wider placement, to overcome these challenges?

Learning within children and young people's services

Learning is at the heart of children's and young people's services, regardless of the setting or context and is related to the emphasis on holistic approaches to the support of service users and their development. Learning is often reciprocal, as the relationship between the service users and practitioners develop. It is therefore essential that placement supervisors are equipped to support practitioners in understanding and applying learning theories to ensure that the educational aspects are effective and appropriately tailored towards learning and development.

Learning theory in practice

Learning theories provide a framework for understanding how learning occurs and can inform instructional strategies and educational practices (Mukhalalati and Taylor, 2019). Being aware of multiple models allows the practitioner to create bespoke learning environments tailored more specifically to the needs of children and young people. Table 10.1 outlines several learning theories and suggests how these might be relevant when working with children and young people.

Table 10.1 Learning theory and relevance to service provision

Learning theory	Key thinker(s)	Relevance to children's and young people's services
Behaviourism	Skinner, Watson, Pavlov	The practitioner develops their observational skills to identify any behaviours that may help identify the need for support or intervention.
Cognitivism	Piaget, Vygotsky	The practitioner can help support the development of mental processes in an age-appropriate way, which may help explore perceptions, memories, and problem-solving skills.
Constructivism	Piaget, Vygotsky, Bruner	The practitioner is aware of how the environment and prior experiences might influence children and young people's values, beliefs and knowledge, and can support them to further explore and understand these.
Social learning theory	Bandura	The practitioner considers the social context where a child or young person may learn by observing peers or adults and modelling their behaviour, both negatively and positively.

(Continued)

Table 10.1 (Continued)

Learning theory	Key thinker(s)	Relevance to children's and young people's services
Connectivism	Siemens, Downes	If learning is understood as a series of networks of connections – both physically and through technology – the practitioner can help a child or young person to develop and learn through these connections.
Experiential learning	Kolb	The practitioner can support the child or young person to see their experiences as a cycle where they can reflect on what took place, conceptualise the learning and develop actions to bring about change, before revisiting the cycle to further reflect and learn.
Andragogy	Knowles	Whilst Knowles sought to identify characteristics of adult learners, the principles can be applied to children and young people as they emphasise self-directed learning, problem-solving and drawing on life experiences.
Multiple intelligences	Gardner	The practitioner considers multiple forms of intelligences, including linguistic, logical-mathematical, musical, spatial, bodily-kinaesthetic and more. Therefore, a child or young person's ability to learn and develop should not be judged solely on educational outputs.
Humanistic learning theory	Rogers, Maslow	The practitioner can encourage children and young people to explore self-actualisation and personal growth, encouraging them to reach their full potential.
Bloom's taxonomy	Bloom	The practitioner is aware of different levels of cognitive thinking skills and can support children and young people to develop their knowledge and comprehension through to analysis, synthesis, and evaluative skills.

There are many ways in which practitioners can make use of learning theory in a synthesised way to further develop their practice. Here we briefly discuss two learning spaces, coaching and peer assisted learning (C-PAL) and communities of practice (CoP).

Coaching and peer assisted learning is a specific educational approach designed to support students' learning using peer coaching and collaboration (Wareing *et al.*, 2018). C-PAL is often used in university settings to help students improve their academic performance and enhance their overall learning experience. The coaching element involves a more experienced peer who can provide guidance, support and mentorship to another student. This may include one-to-one coaching sessions, group coaching or even online coaching. The coach, often a fellow student, helps the learner set goals, develop study strategies and navigate challenging academic tasks. For more information on coaching, see Chapter 4. The peer-assisted aspect of C-PAL involves students working together to support each other's learning. Students collaborate, share knowledge and provide feedback to one another. This peer-to-peer interaction fosters a supportive learning environment in which students can collectively address challenges and solve problems. C-PAL has been shown to enhance learning, increase motivation, personalise guidance, encourage social interaction and improve study skills (Sevenhuysen et al., 2016).

Communities of practice (CoP) was first developed by social learning theorists Jean Lave and Etienne Wenger (Lave and Wenger, 1991). They provide a space for groups of people who share a common interest, profession or passion, to come together to learn and improve their knowledge and skills. CoP can take on many forms, but here we suggest an approach which brings together students, placement supervisors and qualified professionals to explore issues related to practice. Whilst those invited will share similar professional values and experiences, the breadth of members may span different contexts, institutions and sectors. Members can devise for themselves their own term of reference which will outline the regularity of meetings, mode of coming together be that in person, online or a mixture of the two and how the agenda for each meeting is shaped. The community may start out by sharing knowledge and experiences but could lead to collaboration and the sharing of resources. Learning is often informal, but the membership itself can help professionals develop a stronger sense of identity, belonging and commitment. A CoP will require someone to lead the group by bringing together a network of professional, providing administrative support and group facilitation. In the context of children's and young people's services, practitioners may be invited from educational, social welfare, youth justice, health and social care settings, to name a few. One of the potential difficulties of being part of a CoP is how you overcome challenges associated with an 'echo chamber' – this will require good leadership and facilitation to ensure discussions involve analysis and critique alongside other cathartic off-loading to people who will understand sector-specific challenges. A good CoP will provide a platform for experts and novices to learn alongside each other, solve problems and innovate.

Supervision as a learning process

When the student practitioner meets with their supervisor, another layer of learning takes place. The supervisor can help the student take a step back and explore what has gone on whilst on placement. This reinforces the lifelong learning process and a commitment to stay on the learning journey, open to gaining new insights and further enhancing practice.

However, there are things that could inhibit the learning process which placement supervisors should be mindful of. The supervisor should not be looking to produce a 'mini me', where an intentional or unintentional aim is to facilitate cloning through the supervisory process. Supervisors should be mindful that each student practitioner brings their own experiences to the table and can make their own unique contributions to the profession. The supervisor is often learning from the student – and this can be acknowledged, for example, when a student suggests a new or different approach to working with children or young people. Providing practices are within the realms of professional ethics and codes of conduct, it is still possible for the student to explore how they might approach their role, which may well be different to that of their supervisor. There may even be uncomfortable conversations where the student challenges their practice supervisor and these should be welcomed rather than shut down. There is a place for role modelling professional ways of working, but this should not prohibit discussions around different or emerging approaches.

The supervisor needs to hold the adult-adult relationship and set a tone of working that seeks to minimise power imbalances as this will lead to greater freedom for the student to express their thinking and the development of ideas around practice. Treating the student as the expert can be very powerful in the learning process. Giving students permission to explore openly their options and consider what might be best for the child or young person, is crucial. Practitioners can often face dilemmas when supporting children or young people going through challenging circumstances and it can be tricky to come up with textbook answers, even for the most experienced practitioners. Providing the space to explore all the options is crucial for students learning how to start to respond more effectively when faced with new or complex situations.

One way of summarising the supervisor's role is to use a scaffolding approach, particularly when the student is learning a new skill or complex concept. This approach is based on the work of Vygotsky (1978) and refers to temporary support or guidance initially offered to the student to help them begin the learning process. This can take the form of verbal cues, prompts, modelling or providing resources. The key idea is that the scaffolding is gradually removed as the student gains in competence and confidence, allowing them to take on more responsibility.

Implications for placement supervisor practice

The learning and development of the student should be at the forefront of the placement supervisor's mind, throughout the supervisory relationship. The discussions so far about the most effective ways of supporting the learning process will vary depending on the two personalities and experiences represented by the supervisor and student. Therefore, there is no one-size-fits-all approach. However, the ways in which the supervisor and student learn best need to be prominent and evident in the way in which you both work together and that will take time for trust and rapport to be established.

Activity 2

Assessing learning theories in practice
Using Table 10.1, identify:

1   Which learning theory resonates most with your own learning style and needs?
2   How might you ensure that your own learning preferences do not dominate the supervisory relationship and create a barrier to meeting the needs of your students or apprentice?

Learning from the family

The family is an important focus when caring for a child or young person. It is therefore essential that placement supervisors consider how the child or young person fits into their family and what the family may need to help them develop. The family is usually the expert on their child or young person and considering how we work with the family is a vital aspect of caring.

Activity 3

Family-centred care
How would you define these terms?

- Family-centred care
- Partnership collaboration/partnership working
- Advocacy

Provide an example from your practice that links to each of these key terms.

Until the late 1950s, hospitals tended to be bleak places for children and young people. Parents were usually not allowed to visit as it was seen as detrimental to the child, as children would become distressed at the end of visiting time. In 1959, the government commissioned a report into the welfare of children in hospital. The Platt Report (1959) recommended that visiting become unrestricted, that mothers could stay with their child in hospital and that the emotional needs of children needed to be considered. Here we had the start of partnership working, where parents have become increasingly involved in caring for their child in hospital.

Other important documents related to Partnership working and Family-Centred Care are: The Welfare of Children and Young People in Hospital (DoH, 1991), which discusses three reports (The Platt Report, The Court Report and Working for Patients). This complete document emphasised the need to share information and involve parents and carers in the care of the child. The United Nations (1989) Convention on the Rights of the Child discusses respect for the child as a person in their own right. Children Act 1989 (Section 20) considers professional collaboration and information sharing with parents. The National Service Framework for Children and Young People and Maternity Services (2004) recognised that children are different and are a distinct group from adults; as such, they need different approaches and different services to adults. The framework considered that children and young people were best placed to inform the development of health services. The Health Foundation (2012) reviewed evidence regarding sharing decision-making. The concept of family-centred care has evolved over a period of years, with children's and young people's nurses applying some of the elements within their practice for some years.

Terms you may have come across related to family-centred care may include partnership care, parental participation, parental involvement, parental care or child-centred care. There is an absence of an accepted definition, which means that family-centred care is not being fully implemented. Partnership working is aligned with giving choice and sharing decision-making; professionals and families can work together, in partnership, to choose treatment, management and care, all based upon the available evidence and preferences. Anne Casey (1988) first developed a partnership in care model; this comprised the five concepts (Box 10.1), with the philosophy being that the best people to care for the child is the family, with help from professional staff.

Box 10.1   The five concepts utilised in Casey's Partnership Model (1988)

- The child;
- The family;
- Health;
- Environment;
- The nurse.

Box 10.2   The nine elements to family-centred care (Shields, 2015)

1   Recognising the family as a constant in the child's life;
2   Facilitating parent-professional collaboration at all levels of health care;
3   Honouring the racial, ethnic, cultural and socio-economic diversity of families;
4   Recognising family strengths and individuality and respecting different methods of coping;
5   Sharing complete and unbiased information with families on a continuous basis;
6   Encouraging and facilitating family-to-family support and networking;
7   Responding to child and family developmental needs as part of healthcare practices;
8   Adopting policies and practices that provide families with emotional and financial support; and
9   Designing health care that is flexible, culturally competent, and responsive to family needs.

Casey's model was utilised but sometimes misinterpreted, as families were seemingly required provide all the care for their child or young person. Some families felt that they were burdened with the care, isolated and afraid of doing something wrong.

Activity 4

Partnership working
In this activity, we will explore the theory of partnership working more deeply. With reference to your workplace, consider:

1   Is this your reality in the workplace?
2   What might stop effective partnership?

In family-centred care (Shields *et al.*, 2006), the care is planned around the whole family, not just an individual. A definition of family-centred care is 'a way of caring for children and their families within health services, which ensures that care is planned around the whole family not just the individual child/person and in which all the family members are recognized as care recipients' (Shields, 2015, p. 140). Box 10.2 shows that there are nine elements to family-centred care.

Understanding family dynamics/communicating with families

Patient experience is key, but in family-centred care we also need to consider improving the experience of all in the family, whether that be experience within a hospital for a visit or admission, or whether it is having a home visit or in a clinic. We need to ensure that the family feel empowered and in control of their choices when we are caring for them.

Activity 5

Policies and guidelines
With reference to your employing organisation:

Table 10.2 Levels of involvement in family-centred care

1.	Nurse led, no family involvement	The family may not be able or willing to be involved in the care. However, this can still be family-centred care if professionals respond to the family's needs
2.	Nurse led, family participate in care	The family delivers some care, may need support in the care given
3.	Equal status, family partnership in care	The nurse acts as support but the family has been empowered to be the primary carer
4.	Parent/child led, expert parent or child	The family/child are experts in the care, and they may be teaching the nurse new skills

1　What policies or guidelines are you aware of that say you should work with children and families in partnership?
2　What pieces of legislation require health and social work professions to work in partnership?

Families play a key role in meeting the needs of their core components; for example, if a child or young person has an illness or a disability then the family play an important role in supporting the health and wellbeing of the child or young person. We need to consider the needs of the child as well as the wider family; however, a child with any disability (physical or mental health) is dependent upon their family to support their needs. The family is usually the main support for a child or young person and the family is the constant within that child or young person's life.

Family-centred care includes developing trusting and respectful partnerships with all family members, ensuring that appropriate information sharing occurs so that all involved in caring for the child are included, thus leading to enhanced wellbeing and possibly could lead to reduced anxiety for the family, as they feel listened to. Supporting families to be actively involved in their care can lead to improved outcomes and experience for the family. It also gives the family the power to make their own informed decisions about their care; it also supports them to improve their health and give best opportunities for them to lead the life they want. The care is tailored to each individual family and professionals work collaboratively with the family members. There are different levels of involvement of family-centred care.

Table 10.2 shows the levels of involvement in family-centred care. Some families may want to be involved in the care of their child or young person but they may need support in developing new skills. They may also want to have 'you' care for their child, as they may feel the need for 'down time' or feel worried about caring for their child/young person. By using family-centred care, we need to consider the needs of the family unit and find out what is best for their needs. You may need to act as an advocate for the child or young person or family, especially if the family is developing new skills or does not feel confident in speaking up for their needs.

Activity 6

Advocacy
When have you needed to advocate for a family?
How did you support the family at that time?

Implications for placement supervisor's practice

Family-centred care needs to consider culture and society, to ensure that family's needs are supported. An illness-specific care plan could be utilised or there may be core aspects that can be applied to all families; however, these would not be specific to each family. Family-centred care means that each child is considered as part of the family or as a unit of care; this could be problematic depending on how family-centred care is implemented.

The family carers are the experts in their own family life and that of their child or young person. The family is the constant around a child or young person and as a practitioner we may only see the child briefly. Even if we feel we are a major part of a child or young person's life, for example, if a child has cancer and is seen on a ward regularly, then we must remember that we are fleetingly within that family's life and that the family is the constant safeguard for that child/young person.

It is vital that students/learners are able to develop an understanding of how each family they see has their own needs, then the student/learner may develop their skills in being able to recognise what each family may need to provide a safe environment. We need to share information with the family in a supportive manner so that they can make the best decisions for their child/young person and for them as a family. At times, as professionals, we may need to make urgent decisions but, if possible, it is best to discuss needs of a child/young person with the family unit.

If the placement supervisor is able to assist a student/learner in being able to 'stop and look at the family' and help them to be able to empathise and walk in that family's shoes, to be able to see it through the eyes of that family, then that is a valuable skill to have learned.

Activity 7

Who is the family?
How do you discover who 'the family' is to a child or young person? How do you find out how that family normally functions?

Some ways of supporting a student to develop skills may be though 'bite-sized' teaching in a student huddle or by having a golden hour, where students can decide what they need to learn for that hour and then return to feedback their learning. Both of these ideas could be used to support and empower a student in learning more about the lived experience of different families and family-centred care. Ideas for developing student skills in family-centred care could be showing a genuine interest in the child; by actively listening to the individuals; by challenging their own assumptions, beliefs and behaviours and by willingness to adapt and seek family opinion and willingness to advocate for the child and family.

Vignette

Sam is 7 years old and has cystic fibrosis. Mum was with him intermittently during his recent hospital admission. You visit him at home with a community nurse as his school is concerned that mum does not send his medications to school with him and the hospital staff are concerned that his take-home medications have not yet been collected. When you get to his house, you realise that the garden is unkempt, you are asked inside and it is chaotic. The house is very dirty, there are holes in the walls and there are no carpets. Mum appears distracted and is holding a 9-month-old. You see a 3-year-old playing on a rug and you are aware that the 5-year-old is at the same school as Sam.

1   What concerns do you have?
2   Using the nine elements of family-centred care, how will you plan care for Sam?
3   What is your immediate plan of care?

Conclusion

In this chapter, we have considered how the landscape of children's and young people's services has changed in recent years and is still changing at a rapid pace, in response to technological advances alongside depletion of services. It is important that this context is taken into account when the student is on placement and being supported by the supervisor – how do they navigate these changes when resources don't meet the needs and demands of services? Additionally, we considered the ways in which the supervisor can be vital in supporting the student to develop in ways unique to their experiences and context, whilst adhering to professional values, skills and knowledge. Lastly, we explored the importance of understanding and applying a family-centred approach, building on networks and advocating for children and young people so that the work is not understood in isolation but promotes connectedness and wider support.

References

Casey A (1988) 'A partnership with child and family', *Senior Nurse*, 8 (4), pp. 8–9.
Children Act (1989) (Section 20) https://www.legislation.gov.uk/ukpga/1989/41/contents (Last accessed: 6.11.23)
Department of Health (1991) *The Welfare of Children and Young People in Hospital*. London: HMSO.
Early Intervention Foundation (2020). https://www.eif.org.uk/files/pdf/planning-early-childhood-services-in-2020.pdf
Lave J, Wenger E (1991) *Situated learning, legitimate peripheral participation*. Cambridge: Cambridge University Press.
MacAlister J (2022) *The independent review of children's social care – final report*. https://assets.publishing.service.gov.uk/government/uploads/system/uploads/attachment_data/file/1141532/Independent_review_of_children_s_social_care_-_Final_report.pdf
Mukhalalati BA, Taylor A (2019). 'Adult learning theories in context: A quick guide for healthcare professional educators', *Journal of Medical Education and Curricular Development*, 6. 10.1177/2382120519840332
National Youth Agency (2023a) *Better together: Youth work with schools*. https://s3.eu-west-1.amazonaws.com/assets.nya2.joltrouter.net/wp-content/uploads/2023/06/20121018/NYA_Publications-2023_Youth-Work-With-Schools_pdf_for_upload_REV-1.pdf
National Youth Agency (2023b). *Better together: Youth work with schools*. https://s3.eu-west-1.amazonaws.com/assets.nya2.joltrouter.net/wp-content/uploads/2023/11/02113902/NYA-Report-The-social-cost-of-youth-work-cuts-%E2%80%93-Preventing-youth-offending-through-youth-work.pdf
Platt H (1959) *The welfare of children in hospital*. London: Ministry of Health Services Council. https://archive.org/details/op1266065-1001

Sevenhuysen S, Haines T, Kiegaldie D, Molloy E (2016) 'Implementing collaborative and peer-assisted learning', *The Clinical Teacher*, 13 (5), pp. 325–331.

Shields L (2015) 'What is family-centred care?' *European Journal of Person Centered Healthcare*, 3 (2), pp. 139–144.

Shields L, Pratt J, Hunter J (2006). 'Family-centred care: A review of qualitative studies', *Journal of Clinical Nursing*, 15 (10), pp. 1317–1323.

The Health Foundation (2012) 'Helping people share decision making', https://www.health.org.uk/publications/helping-people-share-decision-making (Last accessed: 6.11.23).

The National Service Framework for Children and Young People and Maternity Services (2004).

UN (1989). *Convention on the Rights of the Child. Treaty Series*. New York, United Nations.

Vygotsky, L. S. (1978) *Mind in society: The development of higher psychological processes*. Cambridge: Harvard University Press.

Wareing M, Green H, Burden B, Burns S, Beckwith M, Mhlanga F, Mann B (2018) '"coaching and peer-assisted learning" (C-PAL) – the mental health nursing student experience: A qualitative evaluation', *Psychiatric and Mental Health Nursing*, 25 (8), pp. 486–495.

YMCA (2020) Out of service. https://www.ymca.org.uk/wp-content/uploads/2020/01/YMCA-Out-of-Service-report.pdf

YMCA (2023) *Generation cut: A research report into youth work funding disparities across England and Wales*. https://ymca.widen.net/s/qvjn5hfk5f

Chapter 11

Practice supervision in the maternity setting

Claire Bunyan

By the end of this chapter, you will be able to:

1 Discuss the role of Nursing and Midwifery Council Standards of Proficiency and standards relating to the supervision and assessment of student midwives.
2 Describe contemporary midwifery provision in the United Kingdom.
3 Discuss how to support student/apprentice midwives within community services, perinatal and postnatal services.
4 Discuss how to support student/apprentice midwives within MDT/interprofessional care and management.
5 Apply the role of practice supervisor and practice assessor to practice scenarios.

Contemporary maternity services

It's no secret that maternity services in the United Kingdom are struggling. The Royal College of Midwives (RCM) has highlighted the shortage of qualified midwives for many years (RCM, 2022), with the latest estimates being over 2,600 in England alone. The number of students qualifying each year are barely making a dent in that deficit. An ageing workforce and midwives leaving the profession due to alternative career choices or burnout are just some of the issues. Therefore, it is important that we not only support students/apprentices to qualify but also to be prepared for the challenges ahead. Most midwives (the author included!) would support the statement that midwifery can be the most amazing profession, the opportunity to support women/birthing people and their families through one of the most significant life events is truly a privilege. However, the challenges of shortages of staff, increasing complexities and additional needs of those we care increase the demands in the work environment, cannot be dismissed.

Student/apprentice midwives are the future of midwifery and should be seen as an investment in our profession. Ensuring they receive high-quality training both in the university setting and in practice is the key to this. They will be the person answering an emergency buzzer, handing over care or receiving handover – investing the time to teach them, even on a busy shift, will pay off in the long run. By the end of their training, they should be the midwife that you would be happy to care for a relative or friend – it is each of our responsibility to support them to this end.

The NMC code (2023a) says that all qualified nurses, midwives and nursing associates should share their skills. Working with students/apprentices is not an additional role; it is one of the core responsibilities.

DOI: 10.4324/9781003358602-11

The Standards for Student Supervision and Assessment (NMC, 2023c) replaced 'mentorship' as it had been previously. Instead of working a minimum of 40% placement hours with a student to assess them, the roles of supervision and assessment were separated. There were lots of positive reasons for this including making the assessment more robust as it would be based on the feedback from many supervisors. It is also easier to support with the current staff shortages as students/apprentices may work with any registered member of staff. Under the 'new' standards, students/apprentices work with practice supervisors who provide feedback and confirm proficiencies have been met. Students/apprentices are allocated a practice assessor, who must be of the same profession, for their assessments which should be based on feedback from the supervisors, proficiencies completed and a discussion with the assessor. This should remove any bias from the assessment as the decision is based on the feedback of more than one individual.

One of the challenges of this system is ensuring that practice supervisors still feel a responsibility for the students/apprentices – from personal experience teaching was deferred on occasions where the shift was incredibly busy under mentorship the responsibility was still with the same person. If only working with a student/apprentice for a few shifts, it is important that every teaching opportunity is maximised and practice supervisors need to think of the long-term goal – to ensure the student/apprentice receives gold standard training to equip them for life post-qualification.

The SSSA (NMC, 2023b) also enables student/apprentice midwives to work with other healthcare professionals to gain an understanding and appreciation of the role of others. Many of the maternity service users (pregnant people and families) are involved with other health agencies, whether this is social services, mental health services or due to complexities in their physical health history. Whilst midwives remain autonomous professionals in the universal care of birthing people, they also co-ordinate care for those with additional needs (NMC, 2019). Incorporating the skills of working within the multi-disciplinary team (MDT) is an important part of the training for student/apprentice midwives in today's world.

Reports of failures in maternity services in recent years – East Kent (Kirkup, 2022), Shrewsbury (Ockenden, 2022), Morecambe Bay (Kirkup, 2015) and Mid-Staffordshire (Francis, 2013) – all highlight the failure in MDT working in the serious consequences they identified. Student/apprentice midwives should have placements with other teams within their placements, to gain an understanding of their role and the importance of working together to achieve positive outcomes for the service users. The NMC (2023a) updated the education programme standards for midwifery to include a requirement for student/apprentice midwives to experience differences in leadership and organisational culture by having a placement with an alternate maternity provider, with the aim of having a positive impact on care.

Students/apprentices should be encouraged to take ownership of their learning, whilst remembering that 'we don't know what we don't know!' Practice supervisors and assessors should support the students/apprentices to identify their learning needs. For the practice assessor, ideal opportunities include the initial interview when they meet the student/apprentice for the first time, reviews (previously known as formative assessments) during the year and in the summative assessment – to plan learning for the next year of study or preceptorship. For the practice supervisor, knowing learning opportunities in the clinical area, discussion with the student/apprentice about their previous experiences and a regular review of the MORA (midwifery ongoing record of achievement) all provide occasions to discuss learning goals.

Feedback should be given to the student/apprentice during each shift by the practice supervisor. This may be informal feedback if working with the student/apprentice on a few occasions but should be documented frequently to help inform the student/apprentice's reviews and summative assessment with their practice assessor. There are different styles of feedback; however, the most important thing is for both parties to be engaged in the process (Molloy et al., 2018). The word 'process' is deliberately used; feedback should not be thought of as an end product because it is there to help you or the student/apprentice develop (Sambell, 2013) and as such should be an ongoing conversation. It is also important to be constructive, thinking about the language used to avoid negative terminology such as 'tell me how to do it right' rather than 'tell me what I did wrong'. Also, be mindful that comments may not be taken in the way they were intended. As a mentor, the author once told a student that they were 'cack-handed' as they looked awkward when facilitating a birth. When asking the student at the end of the shift how they felt the day had been, the student asked what 'cack-handed' meant. It wasn't an expression they had heard before and they weren't sure how to take it. It was a useful reminder to think about the words used as not all will be familiar with idioms, especially when speaking to people from different cultures or even different age groups. The author has not used that expression since! Feedback discussions could begin by asking the student/apprentice how they feel the shift went and what they think they can do to improve. Encouraging self-reflection is beneficial for their future practice.

There should be frequent discussions between the student/apprentice and supervisor during the shift, encourage the student/apprentice to document the key points and then the supervisor can add any extra comments and sign the feedback. It can be helpful if this is done before the end of the shift, as at handover most professionals are ready to head home and would prefer not to be delayed by student/apprentice paperwork. The feedback conversation with the student/apprentice should also involve the practice supervisor, asking for feedback from the student/apprentice. This can be a useful way of developing your skills as an educator, how did the student/apprentice respond to your teaching style, discussions and feedback? Reflect on these conversations and consider what alternative methods of teaching you could use. The ability to adjust your teaching style to the learners' preferences is a useful skill when educating not only students/apprentices, but colleagues and members of the public.

Activity 1

Think about your time as a student/apprentice midwife. What were the most positive learning experiences? Identify three to four key points from those experiences to identify why/how you learnt from them.

Think about the experiences you had when you learnt the least, why was this? Identify three to four key points from them.

Reflect on these key points in your own teaching style/facilitation of learning.

Are you the supervisor that you wish you had had as a student/apprentice? Remember that not every student/apprentice will learn the same way that you did – this is why feedback from the student/apprentice on your teaching style is valuable. It is the practice supervisor/assessor's responsibility to teach/facilitate learning in a way that the student/apprentice will learn, not for the student/apprentice to adapt to the practice supervisor/assessor's style.

Domain 2 – 'Safe and effective midwifery care: promoting and providing continuity of care and carer' – of the current standards of proficiency for midwives (NMC, 2019) states that midwives should ensure that a woman/birthing person's experience throughout their pregnancy journey is seamless. They should feel safe, respected, empowered and be cared for in the environment of their choosing and that suits them. Following the recommendations of Better Births (NHS England, 2016) and the NHS Long Term Plan (NHS, 2019), the aim was that 'Midwifery continuity of carer' would be the default model of care offered to all birthing people by March 2023 (HSC Public Health Agency, 2022; Llwodraeth Cymru Welsh Government, 2019; NHS England, 2021; Scottish Government, 2020). This was to be achieved in incremental stages – 20% of women experiencing continuity of carer by 2019 and the majority by 2021, with 75% of disadvantaged and minority groups experiencing continuity of care by 2024 (Health and Social Care Committee (HSCC), 2021). Challenges with staffing, exacerbated by the COVID-19 pandemic and recommendations from the Ockenden report (2022) led to many NHS trusts suspending the roll-out of continuity of care, as well as suspending the current provision. This led the government to task Local Maternity Services (LMSs) with agreeing to appropriate time scales with NHS trusts on an individualised basis to ensure safety of care for all maternity service users (Department of Health and Social Care, 2021).

The benefits of the continuity of care model, for women/birthing people, cannot be disputed but for it to be successful maternity services need to be appropriately staffed.

Learning within community services

In the author's experience of midwifery programmes, students/apprentices' practice placements are equally divided between community, antenatal/postnatal wards and delivery environments – whether consultant-led or midwifery-led units. There also tends to be more continuity of supervisor during community placements.

Community placements are a good place for first years to start. Often the student/apprentice will travel with their supervisor for the day and the journey time provides a good opportunity for the student/apprentice and supervisor to get to know each other as well as the opportunity for discussion and feedback on the care seen. Unfortunately, not all first-year students/apprentices can experience this due to the number in practice at any one time and the availability of practice supervisors, which is further impacted by staff shortages.

Community placements offer the student/apprentice the opportunity to learn about the whole package of midwifery care, starting from early pregnancy to handover to the health visiting team and everything in between! Relating this to the NMC Standards of Proficiency (2023b) community placements start to develop the student/apprentice to become an accountable, autonomous, professional midwife (1); provide safe and effective midwifery care (2); understand and provide universal care for all (3) and understand and provide additional care for those that need it (4).

The COVID-19 pandemic presented some challenges – often students/apprentices were not able to travel in cars with their supervisor and were not able to enter people's homes – both for their own safety and to reduce the number of people visiting. There was also the introduction of hubs – women/birthing people would be seen in a hub rather than the midwife visiting them at home. It could be argued that it was easier to follow the 'rules' in the hubs – in terms of social distancing, handwashing facilities, etc. However, the loss of the journey time between visits reduced the opportunity for discussion and reflection between midwife and student/apprentice, and the learning this provided.

The initial conversation with the student/apprentice sets the tone for your professional relationship with them, trust, mutual respect and professionalism are the foundations of a successful and productive relationship between student/apprentice and midwife (Power and Wilson, 2019). The NMC Code (2023) states 'Act as a role model of professional behaviour for students (apprentices) and newly qualified nurses, midwives and nursing associates to aspire to' (20.8).

Activity 2

The NMC Standards for Pre-registration Midwifery Programmes (2023b) also states that 'students (apprentices) should be provided with the learning opportunities to develop the required skills, knowledge and behaviours needed …'

1 What does this mean to you? Jot down your thoughts.
2 Reflect on the relationship/rapport you build with the students/apprentices you work with. What works well?
3 What could be improved?

Hopefully, you will have considered some of the following areas.

Follow the uniform policy: Midwifery is a profession to be proud of and as such midwives need to present themselves in a professional manner – part of which includes 'looking the part'. As a lecturer, one of the challenges faced when discussing the importance of adhering to the uniform policy with students/apprentices is that they often do not see this in practice. Some of the differences include incorrect shoes, additional jewellery and non-uniform trousers. Students/apprentices are given a rationale for the policy – for example, a reminder of some of the bodily fluids that midwives encounter. Most midwives will have had the experience of an amniotomy or spontaneous rupture of membranes, resulting in them 'wearing' the liquid. Shoes that not only protect the wearer's feet but also can be wiped clean are a must. It is not a pleasant thought that if you wear absorbent shoes you will be taking some of that liquid home with you!!

Be professional and polite: This includes conversations, emails and text messages, with members of the public, colleagues and students/apprentices. It also covers replying to messages in a timely fashion.

Act within your scope of practice: Be open and honest if asked a question you do not know the answer to or are asked to perform a task that you are not competent in. This sets a good example to the students/apprentices that it is 'okay' not to know everything – but ensure you find the answers when this is the case.

Timekeeping: Is an important element of professionalism and as a practice supervisor or assessor you should lead by example.

Activity 3

The following activity could apply to any clinical area:

Think about the initial conversation when you meet a student/apprentice for the first time. Spend a few minutes making notes on the following questions.

1   What do you hope to learn from that conversation?
2   What do you want the student/apprentice to take away from the conversation?
3   How do you view your role in the student/apprentice's learning?

It is useful to have some ideas of proficiencies that the students/apprentices can develop whilst on their community placements (both in terms of opportunities for learning and proficiencies that need to be 'signed-off' in the MORA). This may be set out in an induction booklet that students/apprentices receive at the start of their placements. This can also include some general guidance for the student/apprentice, such as appropriate policies to read, NICE guidance and reasonable expectations from the placement area. This should be tailored to the level of study that the student/apprentice is at; for example, first years should read patient information leaflets to start to build their understanding. This will also help them in their early conversations with the woman/birthing person and their family. As the student/apprentices' knowledge develops, policies and national guidance may be more appropriate, developing their professional skills. Finally, the students/apprentices should be encouraged to find and read research around the issues they may encounter – this can lead to an interesting discussion and is a way for midwives in practice to remain up to date. This ties in well with the expectations in the MORA where students/apprentices are expected to participate in their first year, contribute in their second and demonstrate proficiency by the end of their third year.

Activity 4

Create a brief list of useful topics and resources for the students/apprentices as a starting point for the area you work in – you will be able to add/update these following discussions with the students/apprentices that you work with.

Learning within perinatal and postnatal services

Perinatal comes from the Latin 'peri', meaning *around* and 'natal', meaning *birth* and is usually used to refer to the time from the start of the pregnancy until 12 months after childbirth (NHS England, NHS Improvement, National Collaborating Centre for Mental Health, 2018). Postnatal refers to the period after birth, the length of which is usually 6–8 weeks (WHO, 2022; NICE 2021). Students/apprentices will experience this care as part of their practice placements. This section will consider the hospital environment. Some units have separate antenatal and postnatal wards; others have combined wards. It is important to ensure that students/apprentices receive the opportunity to experience antenatal and postnatal care in these environments. They will also spend time in a labour environment, whether on a consultant-led delivery suite or a midwifery-led birthing unit – experience of both is beneficial.

As with community placements, students/apprentices should arrive with identified learning goals for each shift that should link to the proficiencies in the MORA. Part 2 of the NMC Standards for student supervision and assessment says: 'Students/ apprentices are empowered to be proactive and take responsibility for their learning' (p. 6, section 1.7, 2023). Therefore, practice supervisors should encourage students/ apprentices to identify their learning needs for the shift. It would be helpful for the practice supervisor to discuss these with the student/apprentice before the shift starts so that they can identify appropriate people to care for during handover and the allocation of work. A practice supervisor may not always know that they are working with a student/apprentice for that shift until handover, making this early conversation difficult. However, once you are aware that you have a student/apprentice, try to ensure they can meet their learning goals. Students/apprentices should be encouraged to let supervisors know, beforehand if they are allocated to work with them on that day.

As with community placements, be aware of proficiencies that students/apprentices may obtain in in-patient areas and guide them in their learning goals. First-year students/ apprentices may be particularly unsure of what is expected of them and will appreciate the support. Invest your time in the student/apprentice, something that is difficult when it is busy but is a worthwhile use of your time. Increasing a student/apprentice's competence and confidence will enable them to develop quicker. You may not see the 'benefit' with that student/apprentice, but if everyone does this you will see it in another student/apprentice.

Most midwives remember the challenges in completing practice assessment documents and skills logs from their time as students/apprentices. This documentation has been replaced in the United Kingdom by the Midwifery Ongoing Record of Achievement (MORA). Encourage students/apprentices to update this on a regular basis, especially if you may not be working with them again for some time. Students/apprentices need to complete practice episode records and link these to the proficiencies within their MORA, and as a practice supervisor you can sign these. It is helpful to remember where the student/apprentice is in their training, as different levels of competency are expected from each cohort. First-year students/apprentices are expected to 'participate' in care and this can range from being present when the care is given to being actively involved in the care depending on what the proficiency is. Some universities will be specific as to which proficiencies they expect each cohort of students/apprentices to attain, whilst others will expect 'common sense' to be applied. Second-years are expected to 'contribute' to care; again, the level of this will depend on the proficiency but should require more involvement than would be expected from a first-year student/apprentice. Third-years are expected to 'demonstrate' proficiency and all the proficiencies must be signed for the student/apprentice to pass the practice assessment (NMC, 2023a).

Learning with the multi-disciplinary team (MDT)

Midwives play an important role within the MDT in maternity, as autonomous practitioners in universal care and as the coordinator of care in women/birthing people with additional needs acting as advocates for all (NMC, 2019). Students/apprentices should be immersed in this culture from the start of their training, respecting all colleagues for the role they play in the pregnancy continuum. It is useful for students/

apprentices to spend time with different members of the MDT to truly gain an understanding of the contribution they make to the woman/birthing person and family's experience. This should include maternity care assistants, nurses, doctors, midwifery specialists and other specialists within the service. It is also helpful for students/apprentices to understand the role of the interprofessional team and the contribution they make, this may include social services, support groups and other healthcare professionals. If students/apprentices have the opportunity for elective placements within their programmes, these are ideal places to experience and can broaden their understanding of the bigger picture. Domain 2 of the NMC Standards of Proficiency for Midwives (2019) includes 'promoting and providing continuity of care and carer' and is therefore something that students/apprentices must experience and achieve proficiencies in as part of their training. Following the Ockenden report (2022), all NHS trusts had to review and suspend the midwifery continuity of carer model unless they could demonstrate they had safe staffing levels on all shifts, meaning that students/apprentices were less likely to experience continuity of care. Students/apprentices can be helped to develop these proficiencies through case-loading. This may take the form of following someone's journey from the early antenatal stages through to postnatal care, but could also be experienced through shorter episodes; for example, following someone's journey as an in-patient. The important goal is that they understand the experience of a service user and the benefits that can be gained from continuity of care and carer.

Following on from the failures in maternity services identified by Kirkup (2022, 2015), Ockenden (2022) and Francis (2013), the Nursing and Midwifery Council added a new standard to those for pre-registration midwifery programmes in 2023. This was for student/apprentice midwives to experience a different maternity provider from their usual placement, with the aim of students/apprentices experiencing different leadership styles and ways of working. Students/apprentices would then be able to use this experience as they meet Domain 5 – promoting excellence the midwife as colleague, scholar and leader. The guidance from the NMC is flexible, allowing HEIs (higher education institutions) to decide how to meet that standard. Practice supervisors and practice assessors are encouraged to consider their own styles of leadership and teamwork, using this reflection to support students/apprentices in this area. It is only by reflecting on these issues within the working environment that changes can be made. Those that cannot recognise the need for reflection and change may find themselves on the wrong side of a local or national enquiry!

Activity 5

Please take a few moments to consider your responses before reading the suggestions.

- You are supporting Sophie, a first-year student midwife on her first community placement. Sophie is keen to learn how to perform abdominal palpation.
- Mrs Kaur, primigravida and 34 weeks pregnant, has attended clinic for a routine antenatal appointment. Mrs Kaur has consented to Sophie performing an abdominal palpation under your supervision.

    1 What conversation will you have with Sophie to prepare her?
    2 How will you manage the learning environment?

3 How will you give her feedback?
4 How will you ensure that Sophie learns from the experience?
5 How will you reflect on the experience?

Suggestions for the above answers include having a conversation with Sophie before the clinic starts to find out about her previous experiences, what has she covered in university and how she is feeling. It is important to remember that not all students/ apprentices will be comfortable speaking or touching pregnant women/people. Ensuring the student/apprentice feels comfortable will help her rapport with Mrs Kaur.

As Sophie is a first-year student, it is a good idea for you to perform the palpation first so that you can guide her in what she is feeling. Think about the words that you use, aim to be supportive and encouraging. Given that this teaching opportunity will likely mean that the appointment takes longer than normal, how will you manage the time? If Sophie was a more experienced student, you may decide to let her perform the palpation first and explain her findings to you. This decision will depend on the student/apprentices' experiences, the wishes of the woman/birthing person and your own approach.

It may be appropriate to ask Mrs Kaur to give some feedback to Sophie. How did she feel and what were the differences between the midwife's palpation and the students? It is probably best to give Sophie feedback after Mrs Kaur has left and you may choose to begin by asking Sophie her thoughts on the experience. You could then let her know what she did well and what she can work on for next time. It would be helpful to give Sophie some advice for developing her skills; for example, you may suggest YouTube videos, texts on physical examination skills or similar learning tools.

It is advisable for practitioners to reflect on their experiences – how you would handle the situation with a shy student, an over-confident student, or a student with learning differences, for example.

Activity 6

Lola is a second-year apprentice on a postnatal ward placement. She was meant to have worked with you yesterday but didn't attend her shift and to your knowledge did not follow the absence procedure. She arrives for her shift today, but is late and seems flustered on arrival. The ward is busy, and you are short staffed:

1 What assumptions have you made about Lola?
2 What conversation are you going to have with her and where will it take place?
3 What methods of teaching will you use?
4 How will you give Lola feedback?
5 Is there anything else you need to do?
6 How will you reflect on the experience?

We all make assumptions, but it is important to not let them cloud our judgement and approach to a student/apprentice, especially without knowing all the facts. Hopefully you will have informed the person responsible for students/apprentices (in the NHS trust and the university, follow local guidance) 'yesterday' that Lola hadn't attended the shift and that efforts were made to contact Lola to confirm she was safe. Take Lola to a quiet place to ask her if she is okay. There may be a good reason why she is late, so a private conversation is recommended. Remind her of the correct process for absences. This should include informing the trust and the university in a timely manner. This is part of the professionalism expected from a student/apprentice, but also to ensure her safety.

Once you have confirmed that Lola is okay, draw a line under it and move on with the day as normal. Give Lola a handover of the women/birthing people you are caring for and discuss your plan of care. Does she have any learning needs for the shift? Depending on the level of the student/apprentice, you may allocate her a small caseload of her own, checking in with her at regular intervals or you may have her shadow you. This can be a challenging decision if you have not worked with a student/apprentice before, but it is important to encourage students/apprentices to think about their task priorities.

Feedback is likely to be similar to above, and may include feedback from the service users, any other members of staff that Lola has interacted with, as well as feedback from you.

Your actions either after the initial conversation or towards the end of the shift will depend on what was said during the conversation. As Lola didn't follow the trust/university absence policy and procedures, this should be noted on her feedback, just in case it is a regular occurrence. It would also be useful to inform her practice assessor separately to the feedback sheet if you use paper copies; if using an e-MORA, this will be recorded there. If absence or lateness is a regular issue, you may need to escalate further – this may be to your education team (those responsible for the students/apprentices in placement) and the university. If there were any concerns over the student/apprentice's practice, these need to be escalated appropriately. The earlier an issue is addressed the sooner the student/apprentice can correct themselves. Action plans do not have to be punitive; they can be used for development, as was discussed in Chapter 7.

Reflect on the day. Could you have handled the conversations with Lola differently or did they go well? Were the issues something that Lola needs support for? Have you taken the appropriate action?

Activity 7

You are the practice assessor for Rila, a first-year student midwife, who is currently working on the delivery suite. She has been working with two different practice supervisors over her four-week placement. Both have informed you that she appears to be uncomfortable when observing or participating in care and seems to avoid speaking to women/birthing people about these aspects of care. Both practice supervisors have spoken to Rila about the importance of communication, but report no improvement in her behaviour. You are meeting Rila to complete her first formative review in the MORA.

1   What assumptions have you made about Rila?
2   What issues do you want to address and how will you do this?
3   How will you give the student feedback?
4   What would you do after the meeting?
5   How will you reflect on the experience?

As with Lola's scenario, it is important to try and approach the meeting without assumptions. Is there a reason for her behaviour? You could start the meeting by asking Rila how she is feeling, how is she finding placement and what areas has she enjoyed getting a better understanding of the circumstances. It may also be useful to ask Rila to think about how her behaviour affects the people she is caring for as well as what she thinks would help. Suggestions for this may be to read up on policies, procedures and the care needed, increasing her knowledge so that she can answer questions she may be asked. Frame the conversation so that Rila knows you are trying to help her and not simply telling her to do better.

Actions for after the meeting will depend on the conversation. Had Rila taken on board the discussion, do you want to set an informal action plan to give her specific goals, is a more formal action plan appropriate? Set a date with Rila to meet again, perhaps in a couple of weeks, to review.

As with the above scenarios, reflect on the conversation and what went well and what you could do differently.

Summary

- At a time when midwifery services are facing huge pressures, we all have a responsibility to support students/apprentices to enable them to qualify as midwives and want to remain in the profession.
- The NMC (2023d) separated the role of mentor into supervisor and assessor. Ensure that as a practice supervisor you give students/apprentices high-quality feedback to allow them to develop. Also listen to the feedback you receive from them – how could you be better?
- Help the student/apprentice to identify appropriate learning objectives for the area you work in. What do they need to know?

Final thought

Remember the things that concerned you and how you felt as a student/apprentice, when you had good and poor support. Be the supervisor/assessor that you wish you had had as a student/apprentice!

References

Department of Health and Social Care (2021) 'The Government's response to the Health and Social Care Committee's Expert Panel Evaluation'. Available at: https://assets.publishing.service.gov.uk/government/uploads/system/uploads/attachment_data/file/1019109/E02666664_GovResp_to_HSC_Expert_Panel_CP_514_Web_Accessible_v2.pdf (Accessed 2 April 2023).

Francis, R (2013) 'Report of the Mid Staffordshire NHS Foundation Trust Public Inquiry'. Available at: https://assets.publishing.service.gov.uk/government/uploads/system/uploads/attachment_data/file/279124/0947.pdf (Accessed 2 April 2023).

HSC Public Health Agency (2022) Continuity of midwifery carer. Available at: https://www.publichealth.hscni.net/directorates/nursing-midwifery-and-allied-health-professions/midwifery/continuity-midwifery-carer (Accessed 4 August 2023).

HSCC (2021) 'Providing safe and personalised care for all mothers and babies'. Available at: https://publications.parliament.uk/pa/cm5802/cmselect/cmhealth/19/1907.htm#_idTextAnchor048 (Accessed 2 April 2023).

Kirkup, B (2015) 'The report of the Morecambe Bay investigation'. Available at: https://assets.publishing.service.gov.uk/government/uploads/system/uploads/attachment_data/file/408480/47487_MBI_Accessible_v0.1.pdf (Accessed 2 April 2023).

Kirkup, B (2022) 'Reading the signals. Maternity and neonatal services in East Kent – the Report of the Independent Investigation'. Available at: https://assets.publishing.service.gov.uk/government/uploads/system/uploads/attachment_data/file/1111993/reading-the-signals-maternity-and-neonatal-services-in-east-kent_the-report-of-the-independent-investigation_web-accessible.pdf (Accessed 2 April 2023).

Llywodraeth Cymru Welsh Government (2019) *Maternity care in Wales: A five year vision for the future (2019–2024)*. Available at: https://www.gov.wales/sites/default/files/publications/2019-06/maternity-care-in-wales-a-five-year-vision-for-the-future-2019-2024.pdf (Accessed 4 August 2023).

Molloy, E, Ajjawi, R, Bearman, M, Noble, C, Rudland, J, Ryan, A (2018) *Challenging feedback myths: Values, learner involvement and promoting effects beyond the immediate task*. Available at: DOI: 10.1111/medu.13802 (Accessed 13 June 2023).

NHS (2019) 'Long term plan: Maternity and neonatal services'. Available at: https://www.longtermplan.nhs.uk/online-version/chapter-3-further-progress-on-care-quality-and-outcomes/a-strong-start-in-life-for-children-and-young-people/maternity-and-neonatal-services/ (Accessed 2 April 2023).

NHS England (2016) 'Better births: Improving outcomes of maternity services in England: A five year forward view for maternity care'. Available at: https://www.england.nhs.uk/publication/better-births-improving-outcomes-of-maternity-services-in-england-a-five-year-forward-view-for-maternity-care/ (Accessed 2 April 2023).

NHS England (2021) 'Delivering midwifery continuity of carer at full scale: Guidance on planning, implementation and monitoring 2021/2022'. Available at: https://www.england.nhs.uk/publication/delivering-midwifery-continuity-of-carer-at-full-scale-guidance-21-22/ (Accessed 2 April 2023).

NHS England, NHS Improvement, National Collaborating Centre for Mental Health (2018) *The perinatal mental health care pathways*. Available at: https://www.england.nhs.uk/wp-content/uploads/2018/05/perinatal-mental-health-care-pathway.pdf (Accessed 12 June 2023).

NICE (2021) *Postnatal care*. Available at: https://www.nice.org.uk/guidance/ng194/resources/postnatal-care-pdf-66142082148037 (Accessed 12 June 2023).

NMC (2015, updated 2018) 'The code'. Available at: https://www.nmc.org.uk/standards/code/read-the-code-online/ (Accessed 2 April 2023).

NMC (2019) 'Standards of proficiency for midwives'. Available at: https://www.nmc.org.uk/globalassets/sitedocuments/standards/standards-of-proficiency-for-midwives.pdf (Accessed 2 April 2023).

NMC (2023a) 'Our updated standards'. Available at: https://www.nmc.org.uk/education/programme-of-change-for-education/how-we-reviewed-our-pre-education-programme-standards/our-updated-standards/ (Accessed 2 April 2023).

NMC (2023b) 'Standards for pre-registration midwifery programmes'. Available at: https://www.nmc.org.uk/globalassets/sitedocuments/standards/standards-for-pre-registration-midwifery-programmes.pdf (Accessed 13 June 2023).

NMC (2023c) 'Standards for student supervision and assessment'. Available at: https://www.nmc.org.uk/globalassets/sitedocuments/standards/2023-pre-reg-standards/new-vi/standards-for-student-supervision-and-assessment.pdf (Accessed 12 June 2023).

NMC (2023d) 'Standards for student supervision and assessment, London, Nursing & Midwifery Council'. Available at: https://www.nmc.org.uk/standards-for-education-and-training/standards-for-student-supervision-and-assessment/

Ockenden, D (2022) 'Findings, conclusions and essential actions from the independent review of maternity services at The Shrewsbury and Telford Hospital NHS Trust'. Available at: https://assets.publishing.service.gov.uk/government/uploads/system/uploads/attachment_data/file/1064302/Final-Ockenden-Report-web-accessible.pdf (Accessed 2 April 2023).

Power, A, Wilson, A (2019) 'Mentor, coach, teacher, role model: What's in a name?' *British Journal of Midwifery*, 27 (3), pp. 184–187.

RCM (2022) 'RCM calls for investment in maternity services as midwife numbers fall in every English region'. Available at: https://www.rcm.org.uk/media-releases/2022/august/rcm-calls-for-investment-in-maternity-services-as-midwife-numbers-fall-in-every-english-region/ (Accessed 2 April 2023).

Sambell, K (2013) 'Involving students in the scholarship of assessment', in Merry, S, Price, M, Carless, D, Taras, M (eds), *Reconceptualising feedback in higher education*. London: Routledge. pp. 81–91.

Scottish Government (2020) *Continuity of carer and local delivery of care: Implementation framework*. Available at: https://www.gov.scot/publications/continuity-carer-local-delivery-care-implementation-framework/ (Accessed 4 August 2023).

World Health Organisation (WHO) (2022) *Who recommendations on maternal and newborn care for a positive postnatal experience*. Available at: https://www.who.int/publications/i/item/9789240045989 (Accessed 12 June 2023).

Chapter 12

Supporting learners in community and secondary adult care

Rowena Slope

By the end of this chapter, you will be able to:

1 Explain the learning opportunities associated with community and secondary care.
2 Discuss the drivers of changing healthcare demand and delivery in the United Kingdom.
3 Describe how the Standards for Student Supervision and Assessment (NMC, 2023a) support indirect supervision in diverse placement areas.
4 Evaluate possibilities for learning in different clinical and therapeutic environments.

Introduction

This chapter provides an overview of community and secondary adult care settings, including acute care, and explores the diverse learning experiences offered within these settings. The National Health Service (NHS) Plan (2019) and other policy documents recognise that the health service needs to be reconfigured to reflect changes in demographics and patient presentation and is steering healthcare towards meeting the needs of patients with long-term conditions that may be characterised by acute episodes. The NHS long-term workforce plan (2023) aims to increase the number of healthcare professionals in training as well the number and diversity of placements, including remote or online services and virtual wards. The Standards for Student Supervision and Assessment (SSSA) (NMC, 2023a) provide for learner assessment in these less conventional learning environments that may not be provided by the NHS or based in hospital settings. Future healthcare professionals need to gain the experience of delivering secondary and community care for these patients and develop the skills to work in less traditional clinical settings and services.

Learning within clinical and therapeutic environments

In response to changing demographics and health needs of communities within the United Kingdom, the SSSA (NMC, 2023a) facilitates the provision of a more diverse clinical and therapeutic learning environment for all fields of nursing and midwifery students. The Nursing and Midwifery Council (NMC) does not describe what constitutes a learning environment, but focuses on the activity of caring for people, which can take place in increasingly diverse settings. The responsibility for ensuring that a practice

DOI: 10.4324/9781003358602-12

learning environment meets the NMC standards is with the approved education institute (AEI) and practice learning partners (NMC, 2023a).

Practice learning partners include NHS trusts, independent and voluntary services and other state-run institutions such as prisons and educational settings often referred to collectively as private independent and voluntary organisations (PIVOs).

The SSSA was originally published in 2018 and came into effect in January 2019 and republished in April 2023. These standards set out role expectations of practice assessors, practice supervisors and academic assessors. It defines the learning environment as 'any environment in terms of physical location where learning takes place as well as the system of shared values, beliefs and behaviours within these places' (2023, p. 14). And practice learning partners are defined as 'organisations that provide practice learning opportunities necessary for supporting pre-registration and post-registration students in meeting proficiencies and programme outcomes' (2023, p. 14).

Similarly, the Standards for Education and Training (HCPC, 2017) provide for the support of learners in alternative placements in secondary and community care as well as new role emerging placements (REPs), where there may not be registrants already in-situ and patients with long-term conditions are often cared for. Moreover, the standards provide for 'arm's-length' or indirect supervision in placements like these to ensure that learners are fully supported. REPs can offer benefits associated with empowerment and personal and professional growth (Clarke et al., 2014; Kyte et al., 2018). The range of services on offer provide insights beyond acute medicine which are compatible with nursing and midwifery holistic models of care.

The SSSA (NMC, 2023a) emphasises the importance of 'safe and effective' learning underpinned by robust support and effective communication between learners, the AEIs and practice learning partners. Nursing and nursing associate learners must still be assessed by a registered nurse, and midwifery students assessed by registered midwives, but they can be supervised by registrants from the Health Care Professions Council (HCPC) and General Medical Council (GMC); non-registrants such as healthcare assistants may contribute feedback. However, if learners are placed in REPs, then they must not be delivering care directly and must have suitable support systems in places such as regular contact with a nurse or midwife assessor and a nominated contact with the AEI. The AEI must conduct a risk assessment before the learner enters the REP to ensure that both learner, patients or service users, and other staff members are not put at risk. Clarke *et al.*'s (2014) review of the occupational therapy (OT) literature on REPs found that some students wanted the more traditional type of learning environments in medical dominated settings and warned that weaker students might struggle in this type of setting, reinforcing the need to effectively support learners.

Activity 1

Analyse your workplace and identify whether it is a traditional learning environment:

- Face to face?
- NHS setting?
- Illness focused?
- Institution based?

If the answer to any of these is no, then your workplace is a non-traditional learning environment.

Community and secondary care settings

According to NHS England (2022), community health services are those that provide care throughout the life span. Community health services are important for meeting the needs of people living with complex health and care needs and supports them to live as independently as possible, ideally within their own homes. Not all these services are provided by the NHS, some may be provided by PIVOs. Such services may be delivered in a variety of settings, such as clinics, community hospitals and schools, and include:

- Urgent community response, including two-hour rapid crisis response services
- District nursing
- Child health services
- Community occupational therapy
- Community paediatric clinics
- Community end of life and palliative care
- Community physiotherapy
- Musculoskeletal therapy
- Pulmonary or cardiac rehabilitation
- Community podiatry
- Community speech and language therapy
- Falls prevention services
- Intermediate care services
- Specialist nurses (for example, diabetes, COPD, heart failure, continence, tissue viability)
- Bed-based community rehabilitation
- Wheelchair services
- Health visiting
- School health services
- Sexual health services
- Health promotion (NHS England, 2022)

The expansion of community health services and a move away from hospitalisation and institutionalisation requires more responsive and locally provided services. The move towards providing care in the community has consequences for the training and development of healthcare professionals. This has been recognised by the NMC, who have developed standards designed to support the assessment of students in these areas, including areas where services are not provided by the NHS and there may not be a registered professional from the learners' own field or discipline. The SSSA (NMC, 2023a) signalled a move away from traditional 'one-on-one' mentoring to a new model where assessor roles were separated from supervision roles. Although learner assessment remains located within the nursing and midwifery realm, supervisory roles can be undertaken by other registered health and social care professionals.

These changes reflected the goals of the NHS Plan (2019), which aims to increase the number of healthcare professionals in learning and ensure sustainability of the workforce in the global context where healthcare professionals are in high demand. The NHS plan sought to improve funding, staffing and inequality of provision brought about by an ageing population (NHS, 2019, p. 6) with increased demand on all services including community and secondary care. Consequently, funding was announced for 5,000 clinical placements for nurse undergraduates together with a 25% increase in nurse undergraduate places (NHS, 2019, p. 80).

The NHS long-term workforce plan released in 2023 outlined further plans to increase the number of healthcare professionals in training, particularly through the apprentice route and funded by employers via the apprenticeship levy. The plan provides for 'more diverse and integrated clinical placements' with placements across 'primary, community and social care, and in the independent and voluntary sectors' (NHS, 2023, p. 81). In recognition of the changing demographics and increasing diversity of the U.K. population, the plan aims to ensure health and social care students have the knowledge, skills and experience to deliver high-quality care and reduce healthcare inequalities as newly qualified registrants (NHS, 2023, p. 80).

Healthcare services may be delivered using various communication methods, often exploiting new technology, and this can enable the delivery of health and care services in the community. The challenges associated with the response to the COVID-19 pandemic led to developments in technology enabled care services (TECS), as well as the use of simulation in health and social care training and are particularly suitable for delivering community services. It is important that learners gain experience of delivering healthcare using different technology platforms, as these can require a different set of skills from traditional ward-based environment.

Health Education England (HEE) outlined how simulated and immersive technologies can be used to support the training needs of the health and social care sector (HEE, 2022). It is believed that this will lead to improvements in clinical effectiveness, patient safety, quality improvement, staff well-being, patient experience and productivity (HEE, 2022, p. 7). There are important limitations to care quality with these innovations that must be acknowledged, but they offer new opportunities to contact harder-to-reach populations in community settings, especially those for whom transportation is a considerable financial, logistical and practical barrier. Consequently, the diversity of roles that healthcare professionals can elect to work in has increased and further opportunities have been created around advanced clinical practice (ACP) roles that are regulated by HEE, which has now integrated into NHS England.

Innovative ways of delivering learning experiences in community settings have already been developed that can be adopted by healthcare services and supported by AEIs. One useful model for supporting learners in community settings is the 'hub and spoke' model that preceded the SSSA (NMC, 2023a). The NMC (2011) defined 'hub and spoke' experiences and pre-qualifying students are allocated to their placement (hub) in the traditional way and formally supported to work in other settings and with different clinicians (spokes).

Since the introduction of the SSSA (NMC, 2023a), there remains interest in hub-and-spoke learning environments, which lend themselves to a range of service delivery. For example, a learner may be placed in a dermatology ward where their practice assessor is based, but may have additional opportunities to experience 'spoke' experiences at other specialist services, such as a burns or surgical clinics. The hub-and-spoke model has been used to support the training of advanced care practitioners (ACPs) in primary care.

A qualitative study by Gloster *et al.* (2020) of ACP students and their GP supervisors found that the hub-and-spoke method was beneficial and provided students with the experience of working in different GP settings.

Activity 2

Think about the clinical learning environments available to students and apprentices that you encounter:

- How many of those learning environments are set in community and secondary services?
- What members of the multi-disciplinary team do leaners encounter in community and secondary services?
- What are the common mental and physical presentations that learners may encounter in community-based learning environments?
- Are learners aware of the diversity of clinical roles in their healthcare field?
- Are there any stages of the patient journey not accessible to learners?

Learning within acute care

Acute care is defined as specialist care that is short term and usually given in response to an illness or injury that may be life or limb threatening. Hirshon *et al.* (2013) define acute services as the provision of promotive, preventive, curative, rehabilitative or palliative action, oriented towards individuals or populations, whose primary purpose is to improve health and whose effectiveness largely depends on time-sensitive rapid intervention. Acute services encompass a range of services, such as emergency medicine, trauma care, pre-hospital emergency care, acute care surgery, critical care, urgent care and short-term inpatient stabilisation (Hirshon *et al.*, 2013).

Acute care has historically provided rich learning environments for a range of healthcare professionals and continues to do so, with many hospitals offering preceptorships designed to give further immersion in these areas to newly recruited registrants. Acute services offer learners the opportunity to work within multi-disciplinary teams, and play an important role in professional socialisation. Acute services may bring learners into contact with ACPs and specialists within their fields of practice and provide them with knowledge and understanding of future career progression.

The vast majority of acute care is delivered in traditional ward-based settings within the hospital building. However, given that demand for acute care beds cannot always be met, acute care beds are being created in secondary care settings in the form of virtual wards. These are defined as:

Virtual wards support patients, who would otherwise be in hospital, to receive the acute care, remote monitoring and treatment they need in their own home or usual place of residence. Virtual wards provide acute clinical care at home for a short duration (up to 14 days) as an alternative to care in hospital. Patients admitted to a virtual ward have their care reviewed daily by a consultant practitioner (including a nurse or allied health professional (AHP) consultant) or suitably trained GP, via a digital platform that allows for the remote monitoring of a patient's condition and escalation to a multidisciplinary team.

(NHS, 2023, p. 4)

Analysis by NHS England and NHS improvement bodies suggest that 50 virtual beds could be created for the same 31 beds in terms of staff utilisation (NHS, 2023, p. 3). Although the response to the COVID-19 pandemic was a driver for the creation of virtual wards, these have proved popular with patients and are cost effective (NHS, 2023, p. 3). The virtual wards have been created for patient pathways, such as acute respiratory infections (including COVID-19) and acute exacerbation of a frailty condition. Patients are monitored using a digital platform and may input information and relevant healthcare data themselves or wear devises that monitor their vital signs (NHS, 2023, p. 5). These wards require informed consent, appropriate safety netting and monitoring by appropriately trained staff. The NHS is planning to increase the number of virtual wards to 40–50 per 100,000 to provide management of long-term conditions, such as heart failure (NHS Confederation, 2023). Virtual wards provide another example of a nontraditional care setting that reflects the evolving nature of service delivery and may provide suitable clinical learning environments for learners as long as they are appropriately supported.

Activity 3

Reflect on a patient that you have recently cared for in secondary care who presented with an acute flare-up of a long-term condition:

- How might that patient be managed on a virtual ward?
- How could vital signs be safely monitored?
- What other healthcare data would need to be collected and analysed?
- What type of registrant and field would be required to manage the patient?
- How would safety netting identify any deteriorating patients?
- What type of learning experience would this provide for a nursing or midwifery learner?

Multidisciplinary and interprofessional care

The NHS Plan (2019) emphasises the importance of the multi-disciplinary team (MDT) and interprofessional working when delivering care. The NMC, HCPC and GMC ethical codes all contain an imperative to work effectively with the wider MDT and exposure to this way of working is important for learners' development, whatever their profession, field or speciality. The SSSA (NMC, 2023a) recognised that learning should take place in this context and emphasises the importance of partnership working between stakeholders involved in delivering nurse and midwifery training. These stakeholders include AEIs, employers, health and care providers and national bodies who have interests in improving the learning experience.

Healthcare is moving away from the hospital system characterised by traditional wards with doctors rounds and nurses delivering care to bedbound patients. This is resulting in the introduction of new services and facilities to provide healthcare in primary, secondary and community settings. Whilst some services such as trauma care have been centralised in recent times to concentrate expertise in specialist centres, other services and specialities have emerged and moved into the community. Harder-to-reach populations, such as people with no fixed abode, mental health difficulties and substance misuse issues, may find it hard to register with a GP and may have lifestyles that make it difficult for them to keep and retain information about appointments or be concordant with medication or rehabilitation. People who do not speak English as their first language, or have cognitive challenges such as those with learning differences, or undocumented migrants may face further barriers to healthcare. Consequently, services provided by PIVOs are valuable to reducing barriers to healthcare and address health inequalities and provide excellent practice learning experiences for health and social care learners as they provide opportunities for interprofessional learning with a wider range of professionals. The variety of placements on offer comes at a time when traditional placement capacity is under threat as the number of hospital beds in traditional placement areas have been cut (Clarke et al., 2014; Humphries et al., 2020). This can lead to burnout of practice assessors and supervisors who may have little control over the number of learners being assigned to their area.

Indirect supervision

Before the SSSA (NMC, 2023a) was introduced, many PIVO placements were under-utilised, despite offering clinical and therapeutic services because there were no nursing or midwifery registrants who could offer consistent mentor support (Knight et al., 2022). However, learning environments can be resurrected using 'long-armed' or indirect supervision models that ensure that the AEI and practice learning partner appropriately supported the learner. According to Knight et al. (2022), PIVOs can obtain their full HEE education and training placement payment using the PIVO HEE training tariff procedure (Department of Health and Social Care, 2023).

The long-arm/indirect supervision model (NMC, 2023b) has the following advantages:

1 Gives placement student independence, increases students' confidence in their abilities and their own time management, giving them a good placement experience, which can boost future recruitment.
2 Increases placement capacity as long-arm/indirect supervisor can take on more students at a distance.
3 Allows rotational opportunities for students in different services, giving them a greater depth of experience and knowledge from across system.

The pioneers of role-emergent learning environments were occupational therapists (OTs) (Kyte et al., 2018) in recognition that care delivery was increasingly taking place away from traditional settings. The role-emergent settings established by OTs featured on-site supervisors and 'long-armed supervision' from clinical supervisors who visited once a week (RCOT, 2016). Other health and social care professions began to recognise the value of more diverse learning environments, including physiotherapist educators. A study by Kyte et al. (2018) conducted interviews and focus groups with physiotherapy students undertaking REP and identified five themes emerging from the data analysis:

1   Establishing a physiotherapy role independently
2   Finding a voice and influencing change
3   Developing professional identity
4   Professional development
5   Support

Although participants in the study reported a mixture of positive and negative experiences, it was concluded overall that the placements were valuable in personal and professional terms, but learners needed appropriate levels of support due to the cognitive and emotional challenges associated with REPs (Kyte *et al.*, 2018). The Nursing and Midwifery Council (NMC) has published supporting information on the provision of indirect supervision (NMC, 2023b) of all students, in accordance with the Standards for Student Supervision and Assessment (SSSA). In particular, the indirect supervision supporting information states that:

- 'The AEI (Approved Education Institution), together with their practice learning partners, are responsible for ensuring that students are provided with a range of learning opportunities' (2023a, p. 1).
- 'Practice learning experiences will vary for students depending on their intended learning outcomes, their stage of learning and their area of practice … and provide care across a range of different learning environments that will enable them to meet their learning outcomes' (2023a, p. 1).

The NMC has recommended that students should not be placed in a practice learning environment without suitable support and supervision; should not provide direct care without suitable support and supervision; that AEIs together with their practice partners must ensure safe and effective learning takes place and a suitable person, appropriately prepared, should be identified in advance, during and afterwards to support the student and provide feedback, with oversight from practice supervisor(s) or practice assessor. Additionally, the NMC recommends that a plan of learning and coordination with the student and those within the environment before, during and after the placement should be in place to formulate relevant learning outcomes and how they can be achieved. Student reflection should be integral to this. In conclusion, the guidance requires that people supporting students must have the knowledge and skills necessary to support and help students meet the learning outcomes specified for that placement' (2023a, p. 2).

Learning from clients with long-term conditions

According to the King's Fund (2023a), a long-term condition is one in which 'there is currently no cure, and which are managed with drugs and other treatment, for example: diabetes, chronic obstructive pulmonary disease, arthritis and hypertension'. Around half the population of the United Kingdom reported having a long-term condition (45.7% of men and 50.1% of women), based on findings from the European Health Interview Survey 2019/2020 (ONS 2022) and the most reported conditions were allergy, low back pain, depression and hypertension. The prevalence of having a long-term condition increases with age and reduced socioeconomic background, and the number of people with multiple long-term conditions is increasing (King's Fund, 2023b). This picture may be further complicated by sarcopenia, associated with reduced muscle mass and function, which is often age related and linked to falls and other adverse events (Cruz-Jentoft and Sayer, 2019).

In recognition of this change in disease burden, the Five Year Forward Plan (2019) launched by the NHS explains its vision for meeting the needs of those with long-term conditions:

> Long term conditions are now a central task of the NHS; caring for these needs requires a partnership with patients over the longer term rather than providing single, unconnected 'episodes' of care. (NHS, 2019)

This includes systematically identifying those over the age of 65 who are living with frailty according to a validated frailty assessment tool such as the Gate Speed Test, PRISMA-7 or Timed Up and Go test (NHS, 2019). The British Geriatric Society define frailty as a 'health state related to the ageing process in which multiply body systems gradually lose their inbuilt reserves' (2014). They estimate that 10% of people over the age of 65 are suffering from frailty and between 25 and 50% of those over the age of 85 (BGS, 2014), and this has significant impacts on community and secondary care.

Policy initiatives by the U.K. government recognise that the population is ageing and that many of these individuals living with multiple long-term chronic conditions are vulnerable to acute episodes. As NHS services are reconfigured to meet these changing needs, so too are changes been brought about to the practice learning environment so that new registrants have the flexibility, insights and understanding to provide these services. According to the King's Fund (2023a) and their analysis of Office for National Statistics (ONS) data, the population of the United Kingdom is set to grow by 8 million between 2012 and 2032 and ethnic populations will comprise 15% of England's population and 37% of London during this period. The proportion of people between the ages of 65–84 will increase by 39% and those over 85 by 106% (King's Fund, 2023b). Improvements in healthcare have resulted in increased longevity, but greater numbers of people are living with multiple comorbidities and have complex health and social care needs often featuring polypharmacy.

Given the complexity of patient presentation, the medical model focused on one disease and one system is failing to meet the needs of this cohort. Expectations of care delivery have changed too, and medical paternalism has been replaced by an emphasis on shared decision making, recovery models and partnership working with patients.

Activity 4

Consider a local voluntary service that offers health and social care to those with long-term conditions. Identify:

- How is the service advertised and how do patients or service users access the service (face to face/scheduled appointments)?
- How are patients or service users referred to the service and what are the referral criteria?
- What health and social care registrants support service delivery and whether they are present?

International placements

Increasingly, universities are offering learners on traditional undergraduate and postgraduate courses the opportunity to take part in international placements often in developing countries such as Ghana, the Philippines and Nepal. The NMC (2023a) regards such placements as 'one-off experiences' and therefore do not need to go through a formal auditing process. Nurses and midwives working in these countries and supervising international learners come under the category of 'other registrant professionals' for the purposes of NMC assessment. International placements may be offered at the end of the second year on undergraduate programmes when students will have some experience of clinical practice in the United Kingdom. These learning experiences tend to be relatively short; around 150 hours or 4 weeks and are usually brokered through a specialist company. A representative at the AEI will act as the nominated person that the learner can contact for support or if they have concerns, and the nominated person may be involved in the selection of suitable candidates for the programme. AEIs may decide to establish certain criteria for student participation such as grade targets for summative assignments and satisfactory performance in clinical placements in the United Kingdom. Learners may be allowed to take annual leave at the same time if they wish to travel, although this is usually at the discretion of the AEI.

Learners are generally supervised in the clinical environment, but this may not be a nurse or midwife. The NMC (2023a) states that proficiencies and programme hours must meet the NMC's standards framework for nursing and midwifery education, with an emphasis on safety for all involved and an emphasis on appropriate support and supervision. Learners must finance these learning experiences and costs can easily exceed £3,000 for associated expenses and represent a considerable barrier to participation even if other criteria are met. Learners seeking to undertake an international placement should ensure that they have appropriate indemnity and travel insurance and consult up-to-date advice from the Foreign and Commonwealth Office (F&CO).

The AEI should ensure that learners who participate are fully aware of some of the challenges they may face in countries where care standards and cultural and religious norms are different from their home countries. Learners will need to be prepared to work in potentially hot and humid countries without the benefits of air conditioning or other home comforts that they may have taken for granted. Learners should nonetheless seek to maintain professional standards consistent with the NMC code (2023), even in resource-deprived areas, particularly in relation to maintaining privacy and dignity, use of social media and informed consent. This is still an evolving area, but suffice to say, AEI must ensure 'all placements and learning experiences have proper oversight and governance' (2023).

Furthermore, the NMC have laid down the following criteria for practice learning environments:

1. Students should not be placed in a practice learning environment without suitable support and supervision.
2. Students should not provide direct care without suitable support and supervision.

3   AEIs, together with their practice partners, must ensure safe and effective learning takes place.
4   A suitable person, appropriately prepared, should be identified in advance, during and afterwards to support the student and provide feedback, with oversight from practice supervisor(s) or practice assessor.
5   A plan of learning and coordination with the student and those within the environment before, during and after the placement should be in place to formulate relevant learning outcomes and how they can be achieved. Student reflection should be integral to this.
6   People supporting students must have the knowledge and skills necessary to support and help students meet the learning outcomes specified for that placement. (NMC, 2023a)

Activity 5

Reflect on the learning environment offered by an international placement:

- What benefits might there be to the learner?
- What benefits might there be to the host learning environment?
- What support will the learner need before, during and after an international placement?
- How should learners be supported and supervised within the international placement and by the nominated person?

Summary

This chapter has explored how changing demographics and patient characteristics have led to an increasingly diverse and ageing population. Around 50% of the adult population lives with at least one long-term chronic condition according to the European Health Interview Survey 2019/2020 (ONS, 2022), which may be complicated with polypharmacy, sarcopenia and fragility. The previous medical model based on one disease and one system can no longer meet the needs of this complex cohort and requires healthcare practitioners to be more adaptive, creative and flexible. Services are being reconfigured to meet these needs, particularly in community and secondary care settings, and learners need to experience care delivery in these different settings.

The healthcare professional of the future must be adaptable, willing to work in collaboration with the wider MDT and in partnership with patients and service users. This requires more creative and flexible clinical learning experiences and may include role emergent placements, virtual wards, technology-enabled care services and international placements. The SSSA (NMC, 2023a) provides for more flexible arrangements in relation to the supervision and assessment of learners in a range of clinical learning environments through long-arm supervision models in role emergency and non-traditional settings that might feature virtual wards or be based abroad. However, AEIs must ensure that these learning opportunities are safe and effective for all involved.

References

Clarke, C, de Visser, R, Martin, M, Sadlo, G (2014) Role-emerging placements: A useful model for occupational therapy practice education? A review of the literature. *International Journal of Practice-based Learning in Health and Social Care*, 2, 14–26. 10.11120/pblh.2014.00020.

Cruz-Jentoft, A, Sayer, AA (2019) 'Sarcopenia', *The Lancet*, 393 (10191), pp. 2636–2646. Available at: https://www.thelancet.com/article/S0140-6736(19)31138-9/fulltext (Accessed: 13 November 2023).

Department of Health and Social Care. (2023) *Education and training tariff guidance 2023 to 2024*. Available at: https://assets.publishing.service.gov.uk/government/uploads/system/uploads/attachment_data/file/1148099/education-and-training-tariffs-guidance-2023-to-2024.pdf (Accessed: 31 October 2023).

Gloster, AS, Tomlins, L, Murphy, N (2020) 'Experiences of advanced clinical practitioners in training and supervisors in primary care using a hub and spoke model', *Practice Nursing*, 31 (8). Available at: https://www.magonlinelibrary.com/doi/full/10.12968/pnur.2020.31.8.334?casa_token=tXHycLN5fdsAAAAA%3AK6oCKKNhMqFd_7fHjpuqGjYkzpqU149a6nVjzM_CGhPhpZPti6QXv4fVs4y9fgLwjjfDeh3vrdtp (Accessed: 31 October 2023).

HCPC (2017) *Standards of education and training, London, Health & Care Professions Council*. Available at https://www.hcpc-uk.org/resources/standards/standards-of-education-and-training/

Health Education England (HEE) (2022) *Enhancing education, clinical practice and staff wellbeing. A national vision for the role of simulation and immersive learning technologies in health and care*. Available at: https://www.hee.nhs.uk/sites/default/files/documents/National%20Strategic%20Vision%20of%20Sim%20in%20Health%20and%20Care.pdf (Accessed: 31 October 2023).

Hirshon, JM, Risko, N, Calvello, EJ, Stewart de Ramirez, S, Narayan, M, Theodosis, C, O'Neill, J (2013) 'Acute care research collaborative at the University of Maryland Global Health Initiative. Health systems and services: the role of acute care', *Bulletin of the World Health Organisation*. May 1, 91 (5), 386–388. doi: 10.2471/BLT.12.112664.

Humphries, B, Keeley, S, Stainer, L, Watson, A (2020) 'An alternative placement model for nursing students: Discovering new horizons', *British Journal of Healthcare Management*, 26 (5). Available at: https://www.magonlinelibrary.com/doi/abs/10.12968/bjhc.2020.0012 (Accessed: 31 October 2023).

Knight, KH, Whaley, V, Bailey-McHale, B, Simpson, A, Hay, J (2022) 'The long-arm approach to placement supervision and assessment', *British Journal of Nursing*, 31, 247–247. 10.12968/bjon.2022.31.4.247.

Kyte, R, Frank, H, Thomas, Y (2018) 'Physiotherapy students' experiences of role-emerging placements: A qualitative study', *International Journal of Practice-based Learning in Health and Social Care*, 6, 1–13. 10.18552/ijpblhsc.v6i2.505.

NHS (2019) NHS long term plan 2019. Available at: https://www.longtermplan.nhs.uk/wp-content/uploads/2019/08/nhs-long-term-plan-version-1.2.pdf (Accessed: 31 October 2023).

NHS (2023) *NHS long term workforce plan*. Available at: https://www.england.nhs.uk/wp-content/uploads/2023/06/nhs-long-term-workforce-plan-v1.2.pdf (Accessed: 31 October 2023).

NHS Confederation (2023) *Realising the potential of virtual wards: Exploring the critical success factors for realising the ambitions of virtual wards*. Available at: https://www.nhsconfed.org/publications/realising-potential-virtual-wards (Accessed: 31 October 2023).

NHS England (2022) *Supporting information: Virtual ward including hospital at home*. Available at: https://www.england.nhs.uk/wp-content/uploads/2021/12/B1478-supporting-guidance-virtual-ward-including-hospital-at-home-march-2022-update.pdf (Accessed: 31 October 2023).

NMC (2011) *Implementing the standards for pre-registration nursing education*. London: NMC.

NMC (2023a) *Standards for student supervision and assessment*. Available at: https://www.nmc.org.uk/standards-for-education-and-training/standards-for-student-supervision-and-assessment/ (Accessed: 31 October 2023).

NMC (2023b) 'Supporting information on indirect supervision, London, Nursing & Midwifery Council'. At: https://www.nmc.org.uk/standards/guidance/supporting-information-on-indirect-supervision/#:~:text=The%20safety%20of%20students%20and,without%20suitable%20support%20and%20supervision.

ONS (2022) *UK health indicators 2019–2020*. Available at: https://www.ons.gov.uk/peoplepopulationandcommunity/healthandsocialcare/healthandlifeexpectancies/bulletins/ukhealthindicators/2019to2020 (Accessed: 13 November 2023).

RCOT (2016) *An investigation into occupational therapy practice education across the UK*, London, Royal College of Occupational Therapists. Available at: chrome-extension://efaidnbmnnnibpcajpcglclefindmkaj/https://www.rcot.co.uk/sites/default/files/InvestigationOTpracticeEd%20RCOT.pdf

The King's Fund (2023a) *Demography: Future trends*. Available at: https://www.kingsfund.org.uk/projects/time-think-differently/trends-demography#:~:text=Over%20the%20next%2020%20years%20the%20population%20aged%2065%2D84,85%20by%20106%20per%20cent.&text=expected%20to%20grow-,The%20number%20of%20deaths%20each%20year%20is%20expected%20to%20grow,462%2C000%20to%20520%2C000%20by%202032 (Accessed: 31 October 2023).

The King's Fund (2023b) *Long term conditions and multi morbidity*. Available at: https://www.kingsfund.org.uk/projects/time-think-differently/trends-disease-and-disability-long-term-conditions-multi-morbidity (Accessed: 13 November 2023).

Turner, G (2014) *Introduction to frailty: Part 1*. British Geriatrics Society Available at: https://www.bgs.org.uk/resources/introduction-to-frailty (Accessed 13 November 2023).

Chapter 13

Practice supervision in mental health services

Mark Wareing and David Roberts

By the end of this chapter, you will be able to:

1 Analyse the role of the practice supervisor, assessor and educator within contemporary mental health service provision.
2 Evaluate a range of learning affordances to prepare students and apprentices to be assessed in practice.
3 Describe at least four strategies to enable students and apprentices to engage in participatory learning with clients with enduring mental health conditions using conversational and recovery models.

Introduction

A key theme in this chapter will be the extent to which students, apprentices and trainees can be supported to be proficient in meeting the holistic healthcare needs of patients, clients and service users. The concept of participatory learning will be introduced with particular reference to activities and learning affordances and their relationship to the successful completion of practice assessments. Practice supervisors, assessors and educators have a particular responsibility to understand the nature of communication with patients, clients and service users and how communicative action is deployed to support learning within the workplace. The three-phase conversational model (TPCM) will be introduced as a tool for the personal development of practice supervisors and learners and is relevant to a range of mental health practice settings. Communication with regard to the conduct of student assessment will also be explored with reference to managing students who challenge assessment processes and decisions.

Participatory learning within contemporary mental health settings

Health and social work students, apprentices, trainers and learners are required to engage in practice by participating in the care, management and support of a range of patients, clients, service users and their families. Within clinical settings, the supervision of student learning has been characterised by learners opportunistically engaging in a range of situations through the use of particular clients, as a vehicle for questioning, organising care and being debriefed by their supervisor at the end of the working day (Wareing, 2012). Billett et al. (2004) argued that engagement in work activity can be more than just completing a task. It can induce lasting cognitive legacies, as a learner's knowledge will

DOI: 10.4324/9781003358602-13

be changed through engagement in goal-directed activities such as the completion of proficiencies, reflection and the assessment of episodes of care and medication management. How each workplace or practice setting 'affords' opportunities for individuals to participate in and learn through workplace activities is one aspect, whereas how learners elect to engage with learning affordances is based on the extent to which learners are invited, expected to learn and practise tasks that contribute to the workplace's continuity (Billett *et al.*, 2004). The features of participatory learning include:

- **An invitation to learn:** being recognised and valued as a learner as well as a worker;
- **Access to learning affordances:** activity, learning and practice opportunity;
- **Individual engagement:** a willingness of the individual to demonstrate sufficient commitment and willingness to participate in care and engage with patients, clients, service users and their families;
- **Personal agency:** the extent of motivation and volition sufficient to play an active role in the setting of goals and learning objectives and prepare, negotiate and complete formative and summative assessments whilst taking ownership of personal development.

As we shall see in this chapter, participatory learning is not only a pedagogical approach, but is closely related to the current assessment strategy for pre-registration healthcare students, as we will see later when we explore the assessment needs of Sarah, Dilys and Ronnie. Practice supervisors need to be able to confidently suggest a range of participatory learning strategies to not only enable students to connect their learning objectives to learning affordances, but as a vehicle for becoming proficient ahead of practice assessment.

Table 13.1 summarises a range of participatory learning strategies that can be used by students, apprentices and trainees within any clinical, therapeutic, in-patient, team-based or community setting.

Table 13.1 Strategies for participatory learning

Mimetic learning: learning from imitation and mirroring the behaviour and actions of another professional	**Opportunistic learning:** identifying, negotiating and securing specific learning experiences and new opportunities	**Participatory learning:** actively engaging in work, care-giving, client interventions and becoming a member of the team
Shadowing: closely observing a professional for a negotiated period	**Role modelling:** identifying values, actions, approaches, individual behaviours, personal characteristics	**Observation:** active observation or the delivery of support, care, therapy, interactions; service provision, practice, management
Reflection-in-learning: reflecting in real time; in the heat of the moment; on the job; in the flow of work	**Learning log:** setting personal learning objectives for completion each day and adapting them accordingly	**Journaling:** an informal diary of interesting events, experiences, impressions associated with place and time

(Continued)

Table 13.1 (Continued)

Story-writing/telling: fact-fiction stories that suggest what could/ might happen next	Hub and spoke experience: spending a day with, or joining a team linked to or organised from a 'base' placement	Poster: a form of guided learning where a learner is tasked to create a poster relating to a specific topic and present to supervisor, educator or peers
Digital narrative: video or audio podcast, story-board, animation, PowerPoint with a focus/central message	Peer-assisted learning: students actively supporting the learning of each other and assisting one another to meet learning objectives with support from a coach	Reflection-on-learning: reflection that occurs after the event, retrospectively either individually, as a group or by an organisation

Participatory learning strategies are particularly useful in assisting learners to develop their communication skills and attend to the quality and development of their communicative actions.

Learning through communicative action

The philosopher and social theorist Jürgen Habermas argued that communicative action was characterised by language used as a medium for understanding and stated that social actors have the same interpretive capacities as social scientists with regard to their ability to interpret communication within particular life worlds (Habermas, 1984, p. 15). Habermas regarded communicative action as a means of transmitting cultural knowledge, which led to mutual understanding, social integration and solidarity. An example could be the extent to which health and social work practitioners are required to communicate within the life world of the multidisciplinary team and engage in forms of interprofessional communicative actions, in addition to using person-centred and therapeutic forms of communication when engaging with patients, clients and service users. Videbeck et al. (2009) created a conversational model (see Figure 13.1) comprising of three phases to enable health and social work students to guide their patient and client interactions and as a tool to focus their reflection.

Activity 1

Using the three-phase conversational model (TPCM) in Figure 13.1, identify:

1 What client and care episodes within your own clinical, service or therapeutic setting would present an opportunity to use the TPCM to reflect on your role as a practice supervisor or practice educator?
2 How might the TPCM be used to prepare students and apprentices for formative and summative assessments?
3 To what extent could the TPCM be used in order to enable students and apprentices to come to a judgement regarding their level of competency or proficiency?

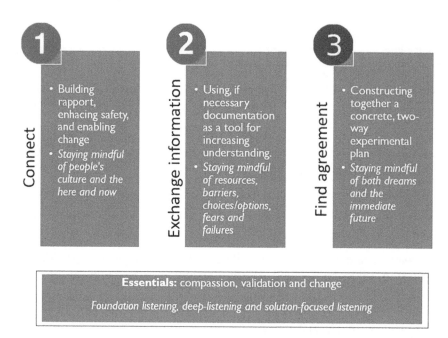

Connect
- Building rapport, enhacing safety, and enabling change
- *Staying mindful of people's culture and the here and now*

Exchange information
- Using, if necessary documentation as a tool for increasing understanding.
- *Staying mindful of resources, barriers, choices/options, fears and failures*

Find agreement
- Constructing together a concrete, two-way experimental plan
- *Staying mindful of both dreams and the immediate future*

Essentials: compassion, validation and change

Foundation listening, deep-listening and solution-focused listening

Figure 13.1 Three-phase conversational model (TPCM).

Hopefully, this activity will have enabled you to see how you can use the TPCM to develop and reflect on your practice as a supervisor and practitioner and enable you to hold reflective, developmental 'conversations that matter' with a range of learners. Table 13.1 presented a range of participatory learning strategies that can assist students and apprentices to learn, not only by working with, but alongside, a range of clinical social actors, through observation, imitation and the modelling of communicative behaviours whilst capturing learning using a range of digital, written, reflective and narrative forms. The TPCM could be used by students and apprentices to explore their level of engagement in participatory learning and to identify any barriers and enablers relating to opportunistic learning and the completion of personal learning objectives.

In the next section, we will turn our attention to a particularly important challenge within contemporary mental health service provision: the provision of meeting physical healthcare needs with particular reference to the standards of proficiency for nursing associates and registered nurses determined by the Nursing and Midwifery Council (NMC).

Physical healthcare needs within mental health settings

In this first activity, we will explore the role of the practice supervisor in supporting two pre-registration nursing students whilst meeting the needs of a particularly vulnerable service user with complex needs.

Activity 2

Sarah, a 34-year-old woman, had been detained by the police following an incident in a shopping centre. Sarah described hearing voices prior to shouting at security staff before self-harming. She has been admitted to an acute ward with wounds to her forearm, which were treated in hospital. Whilst hospitalised, she needed intravenous fluids and antibiotics for suspected hepatitis and arrived on the unit with a dressing to her left arm and a peripheral venous cannula in the antecubital fossa of her right arm.

Imagine that you are a practice supervisor, caring for Sarah whilst supervising Dilys, a second-year pre-registration nursing associate student, and Ronnie, a final-year pre-registration BSc (Hons) nursing student who has the following proficiencies that need to be assessed whilst on the Unit:

- Part 2 England **Nursing Associate** Practice Assessment Document:

Proficiency 9. Provides care and reassesses skin and hygiene status and demonstrates knowledge of appropriate products to prevent, manage skin breakdown and irritations.
   Proficiency 10. Utilises aseptic techniques when monitoring and undertaking wound care using appropriate evidence-based techniques.

- Practice Assessment Document 2.0 Nursing Part 3 **BSc/PGDip/MSc**:

Part 2 No, 26. Demonstrates knowledge and skills related to safe and effective cannulation in line with local policy.
   What sources of clinical expertise, support and knowledge could be accessed to ensure that:

1   Sarah's physical health needs are met.
2   Dilys and Ronnie are able to demonstrate best practice sufficient for their proficiencies to be assessed.

As a practice supervisor, you will be expected to fulfil your role in accordance with the standards for student supervision and assessment (NMC, 2023) that require you to ensure that:

- the level of supervision provided to students reflects their learning needs and stage of learning (2.3, NMC, 2023);
- support learning in line with their scope of practice to enable the student to meet their proficiencies and programme outcomes (3.2, NMC, 2023);
- contribute to student assessments to inform decisions for progression (4.2, NMC, 2023).

In order to fulfil these requirements, you would need to ensure that you were able to understand not only the proficiency, but the assessment strategy and the scope of practice of Dilys and Ronnie as their academic programmes differ even though they are

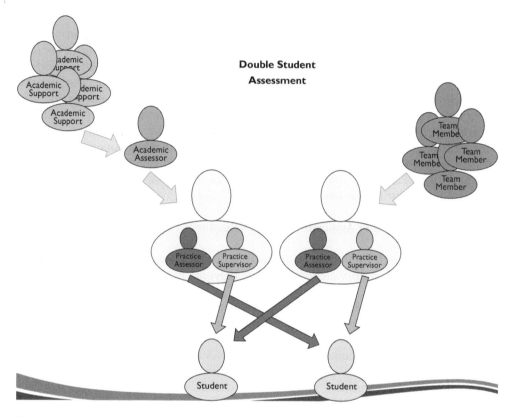

Figure 13.2 Double student assessment.

both final-year students. Whilst it is common for practice supervisors to supervise more than one student, practice assessors may only assess a student for whom they are not their allocated practice supervisor. This 'double student assessment' approach (see Figure 13.2) is reliant on support from other team members, as other registered healthcare, social work and educational professions are permitted to fulfil the role of a practice supervisor. Academic assessors are expected to respond to concerns regarding student conduct, competence and achievement and work in partnership with the nominated practice assessor to evaluate and recommend the student for progression for each part of the programme, in line with programme standards and local and national policies (NMC, 2023).

The nursing associate (NA) and Part 3 BSc/PGDip/MSc practice assessment documents have an assessment strategy that is dependent on a participatory approach to the assessment of practice. For example, the NA PAD states that in year 1, nursing associate students should achieve the assessment criteria by the end of each year via guided participation in care and perform with increasing knowledge, skills and confidence; whilst year-2 students should be practising independently with minimal supervision, provide and monitor care whilst demonstrate increasing knowledge, skills and confidence.

The BSc/PGDip/MSc practice assessment document has the following participatory assessment criteria that stipulates three levels of performance are to be met by the end of each part:

- By the end of Part 1: Guided participation in care and performing with increasing confidence and competence;
- By the end of Part 2: Active participation in care with minimal guidance and performing with increased confidence and competence;
- By the end of Part 3: Practising independently with minimal supervision and leading and co-ordinating care with confidence.

It is beyond the scope of this chapter to go into precise detail regarding the assessment requirements of students on NMC-approved programmes. Both the nursing associate and BSc/PGDip/MSc practice assessment documents are accompanied by guides that can be downloaded from the Pan London Practice Learning and Midlands, Yorkshire and East Practice Learning Groups' websites (see useful links at the end of this chapter). Practice assessors are expected to assess students':

Knowledge: The underlying understanding of the proficiency. Both the theoretical and the practical knowledge needed to implement the proficiency effectively.

Skills: The technical and practical ability to implement the proficiency effectively.

Attitudes: The professional approach to the proficiency. Both in direct care and with the wider care team, within the organisation and outside of it.

The activity featuring Sarah also highlights the requirement for the physical healthcare needs of mental health service users to be met.

In the previous section, we saw that Dilys needed to be prepared to be assessed on skin and wound care, whereas Ronnie's proficiency focused on demonstrating knowledge and skills relating to safe and effective cannulation. The future nurse, standards of proficiency for registered nurses (NMC, 2018), states that nurses must undertake venepuncture and cannulation and blood sampling, interpreting normal and common abnormal blood profiles and venous blood gases (2.2) as part of the procedures for assessing people's needs for person-centred care (Part 1). However, a key factor associated with the application of the standard is clinical context, as whilst the proficiencies apply to all registered nurses, the level of expertise and knowledge required will vary depending on the chosen field(s) of practice (NMC, 2018, p. 31). As a consequence, in order for Ronnie or Dilys to be assessed as proficient additional clinical expertise, support and knowledge should be accessed, which could be from adult nurses employed within the trust (with particular responsibilities for meeting the physical healthcare needs of mental health service users), support from the practice education team and opportunities to be assessed within a simulated learning environment within the trust or university.

Making the transition to becoming a practice assessor is a significant step given the implications of assessment decisions for the student and will be explored in greater detail in Chapter 17.

Activity 3

In this activity, we are introduced to Dorcas, who after sufficient experience as a practice supervisor, has completed her NHS trust's practice assessor preparation programme and undertakes an assessment of Velda:

> Dorcas has been asked to undertake a summative episode of care assessment of Velda, a year-2 pre-registration BSc (Hons) mental health nursing student, who is coming to the end of a nine-week placement in the early intervention team. The practice assessment document required Dorcas and Velda to identify an appropriate episode of direct care involving meeting the needs of a group of people receiving care or in caring for an individual with complex health care needs. Velda was assessed in practice undertaking an initial assessment of Mike, a 52-year-old, who has a long history of drug-related psychosis, who had been referred to the early intervention team by his social worker with moderate disassociative behaviours. The episode of care assessment required Velda to demonstrate skills in undertaking a comprehensive assessment and demonstrate understanding of commonly encoun-tered presentations. Dorcas was concerned that Velda had demonstrated an inability to meet one of the learning outcomes of the assessment, which was to demonstrate that she could undertake a 'whole person assessment' and effectively contribute to the decision-making process and provision of safe, person-centred, evidence-based care. Prior to the completion of the practice assessment documentation, Dorcas consulted with Simon and Kanye, who had provided practice supervision for Velda and had previously shared concerns regarding Velda's ability to undertake a holistic assessment with service users. At the meeting, Dorcas explored Velda's pieces of written reflection, but informed her that she did not feel that Velda had been able to demonstrate that she was proficient in assessing needs and planning care, and felt that Velda had failed to assess whether Mike had been taking or had experienced side effects from his anti-psychotic medication. Velda explained that in previous assessments she had assessed client concordance with medication, to which Dorcas responded by sharing the feedback she had received from Simon and Kanye and informed Velda that unfortunately, on this occasion, she had not passed her episode of care. On receiving this news, Velda became distressed and asked whether Dorcas had consulted with Simon and Kanye to make her decision because of her lack of experience as a practice assessor.

Imagine that you are Dorcas:

1   What sources of support could you have asked for when meeting with Velda and completing her practice assessment document?
2   What actions need to be in place to ensure that Velda is supported to re-take her episode of care assessment successfully?
3   How might you demonstrate accountability for your assessment decision?

Failing an underperforming student for the first time is one of the most difficult decisions registered nurses have to make and requires emotional as well other sources of support (Hunt *et al.*, 2016a). Dorcas could have asked a link lecturer from

Velda's university to sit-in on the assessment meeting, or a member of the NHS trust's practice education team who would have been able to support Velda and Dorcas during what are known to be difficult meetings and, in particular, support her decision-making in the face of an emotional response from the student. Hughes *et al.* (2021) commented that practice assessors find their role particularly difficult when faced by students who regard their performance as suboptimal. In their study, participants reported both positive, destructive and coercive behaviours from students that had led to some assessors 'failing to fail' the student, as the assessor had modified their behaviour when exposed to emotional responses. Hunt *et al.* (2016b) described four types of behaviours from her study into students' use of coercive behaviours during assessment:

Ingratiators: were students who 'curried favour' with assessors and deployed behaviours such as charm, being overly obliging or emotionally exploitative to instil guilt and low levels of fear within the assessor. Although ingratiators had likeable personalities, they worked to sway assessment decisions by doing things to please their assessor, using flattery or tactics such as begging to be passed or emotional behaviours such as hugging or crying.

Diverters: were students who attempted to distract or redirect the assessor's focus through the use of factors unconnected to the area of underperformance. Diverting behaviour may be based on the presence of illness or other mitigation arising from personal circumstances, disability or other proceedings taking place within the university.

Disparagers: challenged the assessor through belittlement, denigration or professionally harmful ways by questioning the assessor's competence and fairness or through an accusation of discrimination, harassment or bullying.

Aggressors: were openly hostile towards their assessor, having received less than positive feedback. These students threatened the assessor (verbally or physically) or employed a third party to do so.

In order for Velda to re-take her episode of care, she will require a 'recovery' or retrieval placement within a new clinical area and an action plan to ensure that she has the opportunity to become proficient in the assessment of clients. An action plan will enable her new practice assessor to be made aware of Velda's practice development needs, which can be remediated ahead of the mid-point formative assessment. As we have seen in Chapters 5 and 8, it is critical that Dorcas documents her direct observation of Velda's performance, in addition to feedback from Simon and Kanye, within the practice assessment document.

Velda may not necessarily be aware that the standards for student supervision and assessment (NMC, 2023) permit practice assessors to draw on feedback from practice supervisors who have worked and supervised students. Figure 13.3 demonstrates how practice assessors need to triangulate their evidence from a range of sources to enable them to be accountable for their assessment decision, which counteracts any accusation of a conspiracy to fail a student, through the adoption of a fair, open and transparent assessment process.

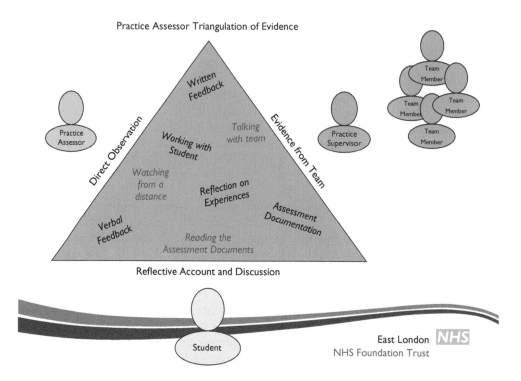

Figure 13.3 Practice assessment via a triangulatory approach.

In Chapter 7, we explored the importance of being able to identify, support and develop students, learners and apprentices in difficulty using a range of strategies, including managing emotion and difficult conversations, development and action planning.

Activity 4

In this next activity, we are introduced to Naz, who is involved in the restraint of a service user whilst on placement:

> Naz, a first-year pre-registration mental health nursing student, is on her first placement in the Child and Adolescent Mental Health Day Unit and asked if she can observe a group therapy session attended by six male and three female young people and a service user who identifies as trans. Becca, an experienced band 6 nurse and Naz's practice assessor, is facilitating the session, when an inappropriate comment is made by a service user regarding the LGBTQ+ community and pride events. Initially, the discussion is refocused and Becca is able to engage most of the group in a thoughtful and respectful discussion until one of the service users makes a personal and derogatory remark, which leads to a physical confrontation between two female service users. Naz and Dina, a healthcare assistant, manage to restrain the service users, who are separated into two quiet areas. Naz is shaken by the incident, which she experienced as sudden and

unexpected. She becomes tearful, starts to hyperventilate and realises that one of the service users scratched her ear lobe, which has started to bleed.

Imagine that you are Naz's allocated practice supervisor and you are copied into an email sent from the Day Centre lead nurse to the learning environment lead describing the above incident, which you read prior to your next shift and Naz's return to placement:

1   The learning environment lead responds to the email and asks that you support the student with a debriefing session. How would you prepare yourself and the student ahead of this meeting?
2   What learning activities would help Naz put into context and make sense of her emotions following the incident?
3   Who else should be contacted to support Naz at the debriefing meeting?

Debriefing meetings

When a student, apprentice or trainee has failed an assessment in practice or where there has been a challenging or distressing incident-related practice, an informal debriefing meeting should be offered, which can be with their supervisor, educator or link lecturer/tutor. The purpose of the meeting is to provide an opportunity for appreciative inquiry using a developmental reflective approach for the benefit of all in attendance and ultimately to enhance the learning environment. If a student has experienced a particularly distressing or difficult incident, they should be offered the opportunity to attend the meeting with a friend or link lecturer/tutor to provide emotional support.

The meeting should be held within an appropriate setting; for example, away from the practice setting in which the incident took place, ideally within a non-clinical/service area where the privacy and dignity of the student can be protected.

Here is a suggested structure for a debriefing meeting adapted from the PEARLS model (Bajaj et al., 2017), which features conversational phrases that can be used by the facilitator to ensure that the meeting is supportive, structured, developmental and productive:

Welcome & Introductions: the facilitator should start with an explanation of the roles of persons present and assurances regarding privacy and confidentiality.

1   Setting the scene:

Objective: For the facilitator to create a safe context for learning.
Task: To state the goal of the debriefing meeting and articulate basic assumptions.
Suggested facilitator phrases: *'Let's spend some time debriefing. Our goal is to improve how we work together and care for our clients/service users/patients'.*

2   Reactions:

Objective: For the facilitator and learner to explore feelings arising from the experience.
Task: To solicit initial reactions and emotions.
Suggested facilitator phrases: *'What were your thoughts and feelings?'*

3 Description:

Objective: For the facilitator and learner to clarify factual information.
Task: To develop a shared understanding of the incident, scenario or 'case'.
Suggested facilitator phrases: *'Can you please share a short summary of the incident, situation or case?'*; *'What was the client/patient/service user's needs/diagnosis?'*; *'Did everyone agree?'*

4 Analysis:

Objective: For the learner and their practice supervisor/assessor/educator to explore performance domains.
Task: To analyse the learner's decision-making, technical skills, communication, leadership, situational awareness, teamwork or use of resources.
Suggested facilitator phrases: *'At this point, I'd like to spend some time thinking about …* [topic] *because …* [facilitator's rationale]'; *'That was a great discussion. Are there any additional comments?'*

5 Application and summary:

Objective: For the learner to identify 'takeaway' or take-home messages.
Task: To enable the learner to identify their personal develop needs and secure additional sources of support for their health and wellbeing.
Suggested facilitator phrases: *'What might you take away or take home from this discussion?'*; *'What might be the key learning points?'*
Additionally, the facilitator may also suggest restorative or mediatory actions, development points, further training and additional sources of further support, such as counselling or contact with a professional advocate.

Hopefully, within Activity 4, you will have identified the roles of practice education or clinical learning facilitators and university link lecturer/tutor who would normally be willing to attend a debriefing meeting to support both the practice supervisor/assessor or educator and the learner. An email to the student or apprentice's personal academic tutor would also be advisable to ensure that 'wrap-around' support could be provided with signposting to university student support services such as counselling and peer support.

Conclusion

In this chapter, we have explored the concept of participatory learning, which is dependent on students and apprentices receiving an invitation to learn with access to a range of affordances, with engagement characterised by personal agency, motivation, volition and ownership of learning processes. Fifteen strategies for participatory learning were presented prior to an exploration of communication and communicative action, which can be captured for learning and reflection using the three-phase conversational model (TPCM) to develop students, apprentices and their supervisors, assessors and educators. Our focus switched to the critical importance of meeting the physical healthcare needs of mental health service users and the assessment needs of Dilys and Ronnie, who were caring for Sarah. This scenario demonstrated the nature of double student assessment processes in line with the requirements of the NMC and how participatory learning is reflected within the assessment strategy of nursing students. In preparation for Chapter 17, we saw the challenges of an experienced practice supervisor transitioning to the role of an assessor, as illustrated by Dorcas, who was challenged by her student regarding her assessment decision. Findings from research into student behaviour acted as a reminder that assessors need to be able to fail an underperforming student, whilst ensuring that there is a triangulatory approach to the gathering and recording of evidence. Students and apprentices sometimes experience challenging and upsetting experiences, as we saw with Naz, who was offered a debriefing meeting, which can also be offered to students who have failed in practice or had other disappointing or unsatisfactory practice education experiences. Debriefing meetings can also be used for coaching purposes, given the explicit focus on the performance of students, apprentices and their supervising educators within clinical, therapeutic and service delivery settings.

The theme of developmental, compassionate and supportive approaches will be explored further with reference to meeting the needs of students and apprentices requiring reasonable adjustments in the next chapter.

Useful links

Pan London Practice Learning Group https://plplg.uk/
Midlands, Yorkshire & East Practice Learning Group: https://myeweb.ac.uk/

References

Bajaj, K, Meguerdichian, M, Thoma, B, Huang, S, Eppich, W, Cheng, A (2017) 'The PEARLS Healthcare debriefing tool', *Academic Medicine*, 93 (2). Available at: https://journals.lww.com/academicmedicine/fulltext/2018/02000/the_pearls_healthcare_debriefing_tool.42.aspx

Billett, S, Barker, M, Hernon-Tinning, B (2004) 'Participatory practices at work', *Pedagogy, Culture and Society*, 12 (2), pp. 233–258. 10.1080/14681360400200198

Habermas, J (1984) *The theory of communicative action – reason and the rationalization of society volume 1*, Cambridge: Polity Press.

Hughes, LJ, Amy Johnston, NB, Mitchell, ML (2021) 'Utilising the invitational theory provides a framework for understanding assessors' experiences of failure to fail', *Nurse Education in Practice*, 55 (5), p. 103135. 10.1016/j.nepr.2021.103135

Hunt, L, McGee, P, Gutteridge, R, Hughes, M (2016a) 'Failing securely: The processes and support which underpin English nurse mentors' assessment decisions regarding under-performing students', *Nurse Education Today*, 39, pp. 79–86. 10.1016/j.nedt.2016.01.011

Hunt, L, McGee, P, Gutteridge, R, Hughes, M (2016b) 'Manipulating mentors' assessment decisions: Do underperforming student nurses use coercive strategies to influence mentors' practical assessment decisions?' *Nurse Education in Practice*, 20, pp. 154–162.

NMC (2018) *The future nurse: Standards of proficiency for registered nurses*. London: Nursing & Midwifery Council. Available at: https://www.nmc.org.uk/globalassets/sitedocuments/education-standards/future-nurse-proficiencies.pdf

NMC (2023) *Standards for student supervision and assessment*. London: Nursing & Midwifery Council. Available at: https://www.nmc.org.uk/globalassets/sitedocuments/standards/2023-pre-reg-standards/new-vi/standards-for-student-supervision-and-assessment.pdf

Videbeck, SD, Acott, K, Miller, CJ (2009) *Mental health nursing*. Wolters Kluwer Health/Lippincott Williams & Wilkins.

Wareing, M (2012) *Rhetoric & reality: The theoretical basis of work-based learning and the lived experience of the foundation degree student*, Unpublished EdD Thesis, The Open University.

Chapter 14

Managing reasonable adjustments

Andrea Thompson, Alex Harvey and Meriel Norris

By the end of this chapter, you will be able to:

1 Explain common neurodivergent conditions and how they may affect the individual learner.
2 Initiate a useful discussion with the student to establish learning styles.
3 Identify what may be a reasonable adjustment for the individual in practice.
4 Discuss the type of training needs might be required to effectively support neurodivergent learners and where to find this training support.
5 Evaluate how to respond to challenges when they arise whilst promoting a compassionate and inclusive learning environment.

   'When a flower doesn't bloom, you fix the environment in which it grows, not the flower'.

Alexander Den Heijer (2019)

This chapter will hopefully provide you with some further information about neurodiversity and how learners with a neurodivergent learning style may be better supported in their clinical environments.

Introduction

The word 'neurodivergence' is an umbrella term coined in the late 1990s by Australian sociologist Judy Singer, when she coined the phrase as part of her honours thesis (Singer, 1998). It can be used to describe conditions such as dyslexia, dyspraxia, attention deficit hyperactivity disorder and autism but also conditions such as Tourette's and obsessive-compulsive disorder (OCD). Neurodiversity encapsulates the different abilities and diverse learning styles that make individuals unique and when it is applied to student learners. Work is continuing to identify and develop supportive learning environments in practice (Stenning and Bertilsdotter Rosqvist, 2021). Those who identify as being neurodivergent may or may not have a diagnosis and this is not essential for learning adjustments (The Equality Act, 2010). It may be a helpful asset for more formal processes such as examination and university submission extensions or disability funding, but actual support can be implemented without an official diagnostic assessment.

In the United Kingdom, an estimated 1 in 7 people identify as being neurodivergent (British Dyslexia Association, 2010) and the most common conditions within this statistic are autism, dyslexia and ADHD (ADHD Aware, 2023). A report published by Unite

DOI: 10.4324/9781003358602-14

Students, the United Kingdom's largest student accommodation provider, found that 14% of all applicants to U.K.-based universities have either ADHD or autism (Shaw *et al.*, 2023). This only included those students who disclosed their condition. Some students prefer not to make a disclosure or may not know they have a learning difference. In another study undertaken by the Office for Students, it was found that 28% of disabled students are likely to defer or not submit an assessment due to lack of support and awareness of their learning needs. Of those 28%, over 11% included students with social, communication and/or behavioural difficulties such as Tourette's, ADHD and ASD (Office for Students, 2020). This is a much higher statistic than the deferment/non-submission rate of neurotypical learners, where the average reported rate is 8.2% (Office for Students, 2020).

Many conditions are co-morbid and occur together, such as autism and ADHD (The National Autistic Society, 2023a). This means that there may be a clearer understanding of the learning adjustment for one of the conditions but not both. The learner is the best source of information about their neurodivergent condition. Spending time discussing how they learn, what types of adjustments may be needed and how their condition affects them can be an excellent starting point for their placement experience. The aim of this chapter is to provide you with some key information about the neurodivergent spectrum, what adjustments may be needed for practice-based learning and how to start conversations with the learners and educators to really provide the best experience for everyone.

Activity 1

Take some time to reflect on your own experiences as a student learner working in a placement or practice education experience. Perhaps this was quite some time ago or it may have been more recent. If you also identify as having a neurodivergent condition or additional learning need, this may have had an effect on your experience in practice. When you are ready, make some notes on the following:

1 List three things that you found challenging about your placements and three things which helped you feel at ease when working in these environments.
2 If you could go back in time and experience that placement again, what, if anything, would you change?
3 Think about the mentor or supervisor who inspired you the most when you were a student working in practice. What was their most important lesson for you as a learner?

Vignette 1

The following vignette introduces us to Aisha, who is a neurodivergent learner with a diagnosis of moderate dyslexia:

Aisha is a first-year student operating department practitioner and is working in the theatres of a local district general hospital. Her current placement is in surgery, where she is learning the role of the circulating practitioner, who supports the scrub team during the surgical procedure. At the end of the first week in this area, Aisha contacts her link lecturer and is anxious, tearful and feels that she is not performing well. The link lecturer is keen to understand exactly what has happened and schedules a meeting with Aisha to discuss it further.

During the meeting, Aisha is asked to list the main challenges she has experienced during this first placement week. Her key concerns were:

- *She felt overwhelmed by the number of different surgical instruments and their individual names. During the pre-surgical checks, she lost confidence and did not participate actively.*
- *She was asked to write the swab count on the board but she made an error and placed the count in the incorrect section. Her mentor corrected her but she felt embarrassed.*
- *The practice supervisor asked some questions during the procedure and although Aisha knew the answers, she was unable to think of them on the spot. This happened on a few occasions and eventually the practice supervisor stopped asking questions.*
- *At the end of the week, Aisha approached the practice supervisor and asked for some skills to be signed off in her PAD. The feedback was that Aisha would need to spend some further time developing her skills and knowledge in this area before any signatures could be given. She felt frustrated that she had 'let herself down' and not shown her underpinning knowledge or understanding.*

The link lecturer and Aisha spent some more time discussing her learning needs and what adjustments had been put into place to support her dyslexia. It appeared that Aisha had chosen not to disclose her dyslexia to the practice education team, meaning they were not aware of her specific learning requirements. When asked why not, she intimated that she felt awkward talking about her learning difference and was worried about how others would react. When the link lecturer reviewed Aisha's individual learning support plan, there were a number of adjustments recommended for practice that may have been helpful if the conversation had taken place before the placement commenced. Aisha was assured by the link lecturer that she should not feel embarrassed or unable to ask for support as this could change the whole experience for her in future. Aisha felt more confident about sharing and disclosing her diagnosis and is planning to schedule a meeting with the practice educator in the next few days. The link lecturer will attend to ensure that the adjustments being requested are reasonable for the practice environment and to give further suggestions about supporting Aisha with her skills-based learning needs.

Now take a few moments and consider your thoughts on this particular student vignette;

- Perhaps you recognise yourself as either the student, the practice educator or the link lecturer.

There are no right or wrong answers, but use your reflections to think about how you would react to the same scenario. It could be a different profession, another area of the care journey or even a different learning need. Apply it to your own environment and consider how you might feel in that situation.

The spectrum of neurodiversity

As you might expect, there are many different conditions that may be considered under the umbrella of neurodiversity. We will not be discussing all of them, but perhaps a short focus on those more frequently presenting in healthcare students would be useful.

Autistic spectrum disorder (ASD)

Finding one definition to describe autism is almost impossible. The National Autistic Society have defined it as a lifelong developmental disability that affects how people communicate and interact with the world (The National Autistic Society, 2023b). This means that some people with autism can struggle to understand social cues, read facial expressions and pick up on the subtle changes in body language that others may spot more easily. They may find situations overwhelming and overstimulating and this can be challenging for them at times, especially in busy and noisy environments (The National Autistic Society, 2023b).

Autistic people may have varying symptoms or presentations with their particular type of condition. Again, like a spectrum, the range of signs can be vast and one individual's experience may not be relatable to another's. To provide helpful learning support and adjustments, the practice supervisor should attempt to find out what type of autism the individual has, how it may affect them and what types of adjustments have worked well in previous settings (such as at school or college).

Currently, there are over 700,000 adults and children in the United Kingdom with an autism diagnosis (The National Autistic Society, 2023b) and only 22% of adults with autism are in full-time employment (Office for National Statistics, 2021). Getting the best and most appropriate support is so important for students with autism so that they reach their potential and achieve their goal of becoming a health or social work practitioner.

Attention deficit hyperactivity disorder (ADHD)

ADHD often presents with symptoms of inattentiveness, restlessness, an inability to concentrate on a task and impulsive behaviours (National Health Service, 2021). Some individuals are diagnosed as a child but others may reach adulthood before being diagnosed, perhaps after struggling with symptoms for some time (The ADHD Foundation, 2023). Some individuals with ADHD may need medication to help manage their symptoms, especially if they are finding education more challenging as a result of the condition (The Royal College of Psychiatrists, 2023).

Some of the most creative people in the world are thought to have had ADHD, including Leonardo Da Vinci and the musical genius, Mozart! Others include famous actors, writers, artists and athletes who all excelled in their field have raised awareness of ADHD. Individuals with ADHD have a fantastic capacity to learn quickly and have a mental energy to absorb information from lots of different platforms (ADHD Foundation, 2023). They are great conversationalists and can adapt their communication skills effectively to suit the situation. They are sometimes hyper focused and will spend time perfecting a skill and ensuring that they are safely able to demonstrate what they have learned. In addition, they are empathetic to the needs of others, having faced struggles themselves. This can make them highly compassionate and empathetic carers, with an ideal personality for patient-centred care.

Dyslexia

The British Dyslexia Association defines dyslexia as a learning difficulty that primarily affects the skills involved in accurate and fluent word reading and spelling. Characteristic features of dyslexia are difficulties in phonological awareness, verbal memory and verbal processing speed. Dyslexia occurs across the range of intellectual abilities (British Dyslexia Association, 2010). It may also affect things such as organisational skills and recalling details quickly, especially when students and apprentices are 'put on the spot'. Students with dyslexia may also have other conditions occurring alongside, as it tends to be a co-occurring condition and can be hereditary (British Dyslexia Association, 2010).

For students with dyslexia, making the transition from school or college to university and professional practice can be challenging. There is a need for a routine and some structure, alongside a clear support plan for study and placement. Learners may have developed their own adjustments to help them in the classroom and often, these can be transferred into the placement environment following discussion with the practice education team (Majors and Tetley, 2019).

In a previous study, dyslexic students displayed a wide range of strengths, including problem-solving with creative and observant personalities (Griffin and Pollock, 2009). Some noted their ability to see the 'bigger picture' and avoid hyper-focused behaviour. This allowed them to find patterns and parallels to situations which assisted in problem solving. They also have high levels of empathy for others and again, in healthcare, this is certainly an essential skill to possess (British Dyslexia Association, 2010).

Case study: A physiotherapy student's experience in practice

This case study is provided as an exemplar. All names are fictitious:

Elliot worked extremely hard for his first-year physiotherapy exams, but his grades were lower than anticipated. When giving Elliot his exam feedback, one of his examiners asked whether he had ever been assessed for dyslexia – in this particular clinical viva exam, it was clear that Elliot had struggled with his processing speed and had repeatedly muddled up clinical terminology. As a result of this exam feedback, Elliot was later assessed by an educational psychologist and was diagnosed with dyslexia.

Elliot commenced his first practice placement a few weeks after being diagnosed with dyslexia. He disclosed his diagnosis to his educator who asked him what reasonable adjustments he would require to help him succeed in the clinical setting. His placement was in an acute ward setting. As this was Elliot's first placement and he was newly diagnosed, he did not have any suggestions of strategies that could help him. His educator was a novice educator and was also unsure of how she could best support him. They decided to re-evaluate Elliot's progress after the first few weeks of placement.

Elliot completed his first two weeks of the six-week placement and struggled in a few areas. The first was timekeeping – he found it very difficult to see his patients in the allotted time slot and also found he needed a long time to write his notes. He was also struggling with his assessments – he was forgetting to ask key questions and not completing objective tests. In other areas, he was excelling – he had fantastic communication skills and devised really innovative treatment plans.

His educator arranged a meeting with the student, his personal academic tutor from university and herself. The personal academic tutor (PAT) gave the student numerous suggestions of reasonable adjustments that had helped students with dyslexia in the past. She suggested giving the student longer than usual to assess and treat patients and also to write their notes. As the placement progressed, and the student became more confident, they would gradually increase their workload. She also recommended trying to find a quiet room on the ward to write his notes and setting a timer on his mobile to keep his treatments and notes to a set time period. The PAT also recommended that the student (with help from the educator) write themselves an assessment proforma that they laminate and keep in their pocket. They could then refer to this to make sure they didn't forget any key assessment areas and to help them perform the assessment in a logical order.

With these support strategies in place, the student excelled in the clinical environment. This case study shows the importance of the student, the university and the clinical educator working in partnership. It is in all of our interests to ensure that neurodivergent students are well supported so that they can thrive in the clinical setting.

- Reflecting on the case study above, how would you approach a similar situation in your own practice environment?

In the next activity, there is an opportunity to think about how to start a conversation about learning adjustments and support in practice. As a practice supervisor, assessor or practice educator, you will be best placed to consider if these are possible and how they might be successfully implemented.

Activity 2

1 Jot down some initial thoughts and then compare your version to the Clinical Practice Learning Needs Agreement Tool (University of Hertfordshire, 2017), which is in the chapter appendix.
2 If you compare the two, did you see any similar sections or questions?

The tool provided may be useful but equally, developing your own version for your specific department may be more suitable.

Developing a reasonable adjustment tool for practice

Creating a tool for practice need not be an arduous task. Perhaps you already have one you could use or adapt? Or you could use the example shown in the appendix (UoH, 2017). The key things to remember when creating a tool like this are:

- Make it accessible for all and ensure you are using inclusive terminology and supportive language;

- Keep it simple and short. No one has time to complete pages and pages of writing and the outcome will be the same using a shorter document;
- Leave space for some updates and changes so that review meetings can make adjustments as needed;
- Consider including a flow chart or other visual tool that explains the process in simple terms.

Examples of reasonable adjustments in practice

You may be wondering what type of adjustments may be needed to help support neurodivergent learners in practice environments. Before we look at some suggestions, it is helpful to consider what may be a challenge for some individuals.

Autism

Some autistic people struggle with hypersensitivity to noise, lights, movement and other traits of a busy environment (The National Autistic Society, 2023b). They may find their own ways and methods to manage this type of overstimulation by 'stimming', which is essentially a way of self-soothing, using repetitive movements, expressions or making noises to help them cope with the stressful environment or situation they find themselves in. Not all people with autism will have this type of physical response and others may use a phrase or repeat certain words in order to help them settle their minds (The National Autistic Society, 2023b). Other triggers can include a break in routine and structure, deviating from a pattern which they know and are familiar with. This creates anxiety and can create stress and worry for the individual.

Dyslexia

Dyslexic individuals or those who have a sub-type such as speed processing disorder or visual stress, may find time management and self-organisation more challenging at times (British Dyslexia Association, 2010). There may be difficulties taking notes at speed or recalling information quickly and the learner may find it more challenging to answer questions on the spot. Many people who have or suspect they have dyslexia will have their own coping strategies and methods for managing different situations but by recognising and respecting the differences in learning technique, adjustments can be implemented without much disruption to the routine.

Putting reasonable adjustments in place should be part of their induction and welcome to the department. The initial conversations should highlight their personal areas of strength and what they feel most confident doing, followed by a discussion about learning styles. Asking a student how they learn is very important, as this will become the basis for the type of mentor or supervisor best suited to supporting their development. Figure 14.1 shows some of the different learning styles that you may come across during your conversations.

VARK is an acronym that refers to the four types of learning styles: visual, auditory, reading/writing preference, and kinesthetic (Fleming, 1995). This may be a helpful tool for practice supervisors and mentors to use when discussing individual learning styles.

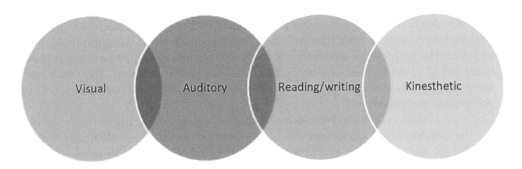

Figure 14.1 VARK learning styles.

1 **Visual learning style**: Learners who identify within this particular group usually learn by seeing and watching what is happening, often being able to recall details of images and actions during a demonstration. Visual learners retain information and key skills from sight and prefer to watch an example before attempting something on their own. (Fleming, 1987 as cited in Prithishkumar and Michael, 2014).

2 **Auditory learning style**: These learners are more comfortable listening to information that may be passed via a lecture or teaching session delivered in practice. They can store the facts and details more easily by listening than by doing as their memory retention allows them to recall details taught verbally (Fleming, 1987 as cited in Prithishkumar and Michael, 2014).

3 **Reading/writing style:** These learners absorb many forms of written information and have a highly developed linguistic skill as a result of being able to read and retain details. Learners may seek out opportunities to learn from textbooks, websites, journals and other forms of written text. They are often confident speakers and contribute their ideas verbally and in writing (Fleming, 1987 as cited in Prithishkumar and Michael, 2014).

4 **Kinaesthetic learning style:** These learners enjoy active participation during hands-on teaching. They are best suited to practical sessions such as simulated learning, demonstrations and opportunities to try for themselves. Sometimes this type of learning style co-exists with the visual learner as the two can be similar in certain aspects but essentially the learner feels most comfortable in situations where they can carry out practical tasks (Fleming, 1987 as cited in Prithishkumar and Michael, 2014).

Holding a conversation about adjustments

There are many potential ways to adjust and modify the workplace for the benefit of the learner. Perhaps you will find the following suggestions helpful for your initial conversations:

- When you first meet your learner, you may or may not be aware of any particular needs and, therefore, an informal chat is recommended as a good starting point.
- The purpose of this conversation is twofold. Firstly, to provide the learner with information about the placement environment, schedule, policies and general daily routines. Secondly, to establish if the learner identifies as being neurodivergent or considers themselves to have a specific learning difference.

- Depending on the information you have been given, you can begin to formulate a plan that provides both supportive and realistic targets for the placement.
- Ask the learner which areas they feel most anxious about and what adjustments they feel would be helpful. For example, a learner who has dyslexia may be anxious about being asked to read aloud in a group or write information at speed. They may have some adjustments in mind that can help them feel less anxious and provide a workable solution for the placement.
- Once you have established the areas that may cause some anxiety or difficulty for the learner, start to discuss the adjustments that can be realistically implemented by that particular placement team. It can be tempting to offer solutions that will make the learner feel more at ease, but these also need to be manageable for the placement team who will be supporting the student. It is best to be honest about what can and cannot be facilitated so that everyone is able to participate fully.
- The adjustments should be documented, reviewed and added to the learner's practice assessment log or ePad. This will ensure that the information is accessible to whoever is supporting the student on any given day.
- Always follow up the success of the adjustments after a specified period of time. This should be an agreed timeframe that everyone is aware of. If issues arise before that time, meetings can be arranged at any stage to address the matter and, hopefully, find a workable solution.

When completing a reasonable adjustment plan, it can be helpful to remember the following (Figure 14.2).

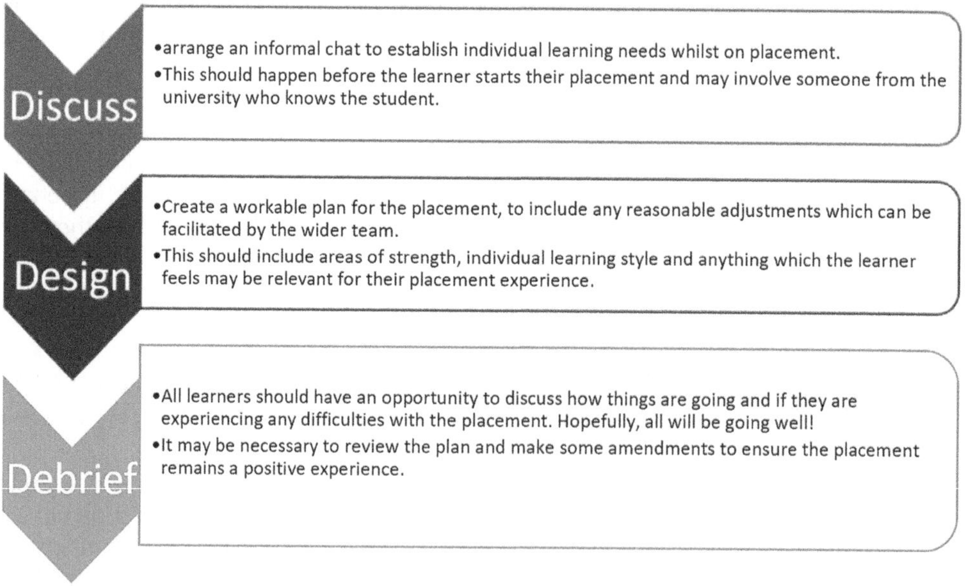

Discuss
- arrange an informal chat to establish individual learning needs whilst on placement.
- This should happen before the learner starts their placement and may involve someone from the university who knows the student.

Design
- Create a workable plan for the placement, to include any reasonable adjustments which can be facilitated by the wider team.
- This should include areas of strength, individual learning style and anything which the learner feels may be relevant for their placement experience.

Debrief
- All learners should have an opportunity to discuss how things are going and if they are experiencing any difficulties with the placement. Hopefully, all will be going well!
- It may be necessary to review the plan and make some amendments to ensure the placement remains a positive experience.

Figure 14.2 Using discuss, design, debrief to plan reasonable adjustments.

Supporting students with dyslexia on practice placements

In order to support students with dyslexia in the transition from university to placement, a number of short conversations were conducted by the authors with students and practice supervisors who either have dyslexia or have experience supervising those with dyslexia. The conversations highlighted the key points they believed supported their success. Table 14.1 contains a summary of the main 'takeaway' messages.

Table 14.1 Student perspectives on support

Student advice
Know yourself and what strategies work best for you. Be prepared to discuss these with your supervisor – you know yourself better than anyone. If you feel comfortable, approach this even before you start your placement or at the very start.
Remember that dyslexia is very common, it is likely that your supervisor is familiar with it.
Be prepared for a large amount of data processing – know your strategies in advance whether that is writing short notes or having mini-breaks.
In some settings you move from one patient to another – discuss with your supervisor about having short breaks in between to note down key points so you don't have hold details in your mind.
Have a small notebook that fits into your uniform pocket, or cue cards for key information e.g. simple things like locked room codes.
In advance of seeing patients, spend some time familiarising yourself with the assessment protocols in your area – note down key prompts to help you work through it logically and in a timely manner.
If helpful, ask your supervisor for the overall plan for the day.
Try to break up the tasks into manageable chunks – that will help with planning and a sense of accomplishment.
Find tools to help you summarise patients for handover e.g. SBAR – situation, background, assessment, recommendation. Write brief notes for each patient to keep you on track.
Adapt your strategies to the environment you are in. E.g. if it is noisy, try to find a quiet corner to help with focus.
You may have to work harder initially but with familiarity this settles.
With electronic notes use inbuilt facilities – such as spell-check and also self-populating assessment forms to save too much writing.
If your working memory is impacted then ask your supervisor to write brief feedback or summarise on Post-It notes – this allows you to go back and review later.
Use audio-functions so text such as relevant articles can be listened to rather than read.
Have personal systems to support time-keeping such as a silent timer in your pocket. This will help you self-manage.
Stay calm – while potentially overwhelming at first, it will get easier.

(Continued)

Table 14.1 (Continued)

Don't be surprised if you thrive in the clinical environment – you have many strengths that will shine in this setting such as problem solving and pattern recognition.
You may not require any adjustments, but being open at the start may still be helpful.
Do not be afraid to challenge negative stereotypes of dyslexia – you know what you can offer.
Supervisors are far more accommodating then you may think. Be open with them so they know how to support.

Table 14.2 Supervisor perspectives on support

Supervisor advice
How you learn is really important to identify to maximise your potential on placement – share this with your supervisor.
It is worth informing the placement in advance of your learning strategies and needs to support planning.
Adjustments are possible, such as number of patients, style of learning and working area.
With the mix of environments, including virtual, different settings can throw up different challenges. If issues arise, discuss these early so you can problem-solve with your supervisor.
Some of the best students are ones with specific learning disabilities. They have in the past re-designed assessment forms which have supported other student learning.
Every student needs will be different, so even when supervisors have experience with students with dyslexia they do need to understand you.
People with dyslexia are often very effective holistic problem-solvers – this is a vital asset in healthcare.

In Table 14.2, supervisors shared their own perspectives on supporting students with dyslexia.

If you have had a student with dyslexia in the past, perhaps review this list and consider how many of the key messages sound familiar or indeed how many you could consider to implement in the future.

The main message from students and supervisors was communication – to share needs and strategies early to promote success in the specific environment of that placement. Do be aware that early in the student's pathway they may still be discovering their strategies as applied to the clinical environment, so reflection at strategic points in the placement to review what has worked and what has not will not only support this placement but also their development in the future.

Troubleshooting

There are likely to be occasions when some problems arise with the placement or the adjustments being implemented. This can be due to a number of things, but most commonly:

- Lack of communication between the learner, the practice team and the university. The documentation should always be supported with a conversation and a brief handover (with consent from the learner) to ensure continuity.
- The adjustments may not be 'reasonable' despite having seemed suitable when they were initially discussed. Sometimes the plan may need to be updated so reflect what can actually be supported in that particular area. For example, the adjustments may allow a leaner to use a voice-recording device to take their own notes at a later time but consent may not be given by the team or the service user. This would limit the effectiveness of this particular adjustment and a different option would be necessary.
- The learner may have experienced some interpersonal difficulties with certain team members. This can happen at any point and with any team. The best solution is to set professional expectations from the beginning and ensure that both the learner and the team are aware of their own roles within the group. The most important thing is that the learner has someone to approach for support if things are becoming difficult or they simply need to offload their thoughts.
- At times, the wider team may feel overwhelmed with the demands of being both practitioner and supervisor/mentor. This is not uncommon and is often exacerbated by staffing shortages, poor physical or mental health or low team morale. For the lead educator or whoever has educational oversight, this can be challenging to manage. It may be helpful to allocate learners with those staff who feel more able to provide some continuity for the learner rather than force a that which is likely to face problems further into the placement. Not everyone will be able to provide supervision all the time and it is better to take a break, recharge and come back to the role when you are more motivated and energised.

Training to support reasonable adjustments

Each NHS trust or employing agency may provide training for you as part of their induction or annual mandatory updates. There may also be some external training opportunities that offer a more structured programme for continuing professional development or accreditation for study pathways. Please see the chapter appendix for a list of online resources and helpful training links that are accessible to everyone with an interest in neurodiversity.

There are also other ways to access information and training opportunities including:

- **Online videos:** There are many videos available online that provide a wealth of information on all sorts of neurodivergent conditions. There are videos from the perspective of the neurodivergent individuals, their carers, family, healthcare professionals and friends. The videos are short and may be an easier way to gain some insight into this spectrum of conditions.
- **Websites:** Each neurodivergent condition has a range of website information and an associated society page. These are valuable resources and easily accessed if you would like to find out more about a specific condition.
- **Community groups and support networks:** Find out what local groups are available nearby in the community. This sort of information is usually accessible through GP practice, community centres, social clubs, schools and colleges. Why not attend a

group and ask if you can listen and gather some further insight and information to help you in practice? The content is likely to be very relatable to your working environment and having an opportunity to hear directly from others is very valuable.

Conclusion

We hope this chapter has been helpful in highlighting the spectrum of neurodivergent conditions and considering how some of them affect a learner in practice. Having a better understanding of neurodivergent learning styles, strengths and adjustments will allow you to provide a supportive and compassionate working environment for all learners. It can take some time to filter changes and implement new ways of working, but take the first step and the rest will follow!

References

ADHD Aware (2023) *What is neurodiversity?* Available online at: https://adhdaware.org.uk/what-is-adhd/neurodiversity-and-other-conditions/ (accessed Nov 2023).

British Dyslexia Association (2010) *What is dyslexia?* Available at: https://www.bdadyslexia.org.uk/dyslexia/about-dyslexia/what-is-dyslexia#:~:text=Dyslexia%20is%20a%20learning%20difficulty,the%20range%20of%20intellectual%20abilities (accessed Nov 2023).

Equality Act (2010) *c.15, s.20 adjustments for disabled persons.* Available at: https://www.legislation.gov.uk/ukpga/2010/15/section/20 (accessed Nov 2023).

Fleming, ND (1995) I'm different; not dumb. Modes of presentation (Vark) In the tertiary classroom. In A Zelmer (ed.), *Research and development in higher education.* Proceedings of the 1995 Annual Conference of the Higher Education and Research Development Society of Australia (HERDSA) (pp. 308–313).

Griffin E, Pollak D (2009) *Student experiences of neurodiversity in higher education: Insights from the BRAINHE project,* Student Services, De Montfort University, Leicester, UK Published online in Wiley InterScience (www.interscience.wiley.com). DOI: 10.1002/dys.383

Major, R, Tetley, J (2019) 'Recognising, managing and supporting dyslexia beyond registration: The lived experiences of qualified nurses and nurse academics', *Nurse Education Practice, 37,* pp. 146–152. DOI: 10.1016/j.nepr.2019.01.005. Epub 2019 Jan 25. PMID: 31003874.

National Health Service (2021) *Attention deficit hyperactivity disorder: Symptoms.* Available at: https://www.nhs.uk/conditions/attention-deficit-hyperactivity-disorder-adhd/symptoms/ (accessed Oct 2023).

Office for National Statistics (2021) *Outcomes for disabled people in the UK: 2020.* Available at: https://www.autism.org.uk/what-we-do/news/new-data-on-the-autism-employment-gap

Office for Students (2020) *Coronavirus briefing note: Disabled students.* Note 8 available at: https://www.officeforstudents.org.uk/media/8f61cef7-4cf7-480a-8f73-3e6c51b05e54/coronavirus-briefing-note-disabled-students.pdf (accessed Oct 2023).

Prithishkumar, IJ, Michael, SA (2014) 'Understanding your student: Using the VARK model', *Journal of Postgraduate Medicine, 60* (2), pp. 183–186. DOI: 10.4103/0022-3859.132337. PMID: 24823519.

Shaw, J et al. (2023) *An asset, not a problem: Meeting the needs of neurodivergent students, unite students.* Available at: https://www.unitegroup.com/wp-content/uploads/2023/03/Neurodivergent-students_report_Unite-Students.pdf (accessed Nov 2023).

Singer, J (1998). Odd people in: The birth of community amongst people on the "autistic spectrum": A personal exploration of a new social movement based on neurological diversity.

Stenning, A, Bertilsdotter Rosqvist, H (2021) 'Neurodiversity studies: Mapping out possibilities of a new critical paradigm', *Disability & Society, 36* (9), pp. 1532–1537, DOI: 10.1080/09687599.2021.1919503

The ADHD Foundation (2023) *Teaching and managing students with ADHD.* Available at: https://www.adhdfoundation.org.uk/wp-content/uploads/2022/03/Teaching-and-Managing-Students-with-ADHD.pdf (accessed Nov 2023).

The National Autistic Society (2023a) *Related conditions, a guide for all audiences*. Available at: https://www.autism.org.uk/advice-and-guidance/topics/related-conditions/related-conditions/all-audiences

The National Autistic Society (2023b) *What is autism?* Available at: https://www.autism.org.uk/advice-and-guidance/what-is-autism

The Royal College of Psychiatrists (2023) *ADHD in adults*. Available at: https://www.rcpsych.ac.uk/mental-health/mental-illnesses-and-mental-health-problems/adhd-in-adults (accessed Nov 2023).

UoH (2017) *Clinical practice learning needs agreement*. Hatfield: University of Hertfordshire.

Appendix 1: Clinical practice learning needs agreement template

This was developed following an original idea by colleagues from the University of Hertfordshire and implemented across our healthcare courses at the University of Bedfordshire in 2017. It continues to be reviewed and utilised as a tool for aiding discussions about reasonable adjustments.

Clinical practice learning needs agreement

This document is designed to assist practice assessors, practice supervisors, mentors and clinical educators (as appropriate) to make reasonable adjustments in practice for students with specific learning disorders (SpLDs). It may be used for those students who disclose a SpLD and give consent for their learning needs to be shared with relevant mentors.

Please complete the following sections:

Student Name ....

Student ID number ....

Placement Location ....

Named Practice Supervisor ....

Named Practice Assessor ....

Named Mentor ....

Named Clinical Educator ....

PART A – Background and SpLD awareness: Student to complete
What SpLD/SpLDs do you have and when was this recognised and/or diagnosed?

Can you tell us a little more about how your SpLD affects you?

What methods and styles of learning best suit your individual needs?

PART B – Reasonable Adjustments (if any): Practice Educator/Supervisor/Assessor/Mentor to complete

What adjustments are needed in the clinical practice environment?

Are these adjustments reasonable and safe for the student, the staff and the patients?

Consent to information sharing:

I hereby give my consent for details of my SpLD(s) to be shared with relevant staff members during this clinical placement. I understand that I may change the level of disclosure at any stage during my placement by contacting, in writing, my clinical educator or student support at the university.

Signed (student) ....

Date ....

Signed (Practice Educator) ....

Date ....

Signed (Link Lecturer) ....

Date: ....

In line with the Statement for Disability Disclosure, the University of Bedfordshire has a detailed and robust system for ensuring students are cleared for clinical practice.

Please be assured that all students regardless of SpLD status will have been subject to Occupational Health Clearance, which will include risk management of individual medical and learning needs.

If you have a specific concern about the safety of a student whilst working in practice, please make contact with the named personal academic tutor (PAT) in the first instance. They can assist you with further support and guidance.

Appendix 2: Links to some free online training

1   The Open University provide a free course on autism, which can be accessed here:
     https://www.open.edu/openlearn/mod/oucontent/view.php?id=66946

2   The Open University also provide this free course on understanding ADHD:
     https://www.open.edu/openlearn/health-sports-psychology/understanding-adhd/
     content-section-0?active-tab=description-tab

3   Exceptional Individuals provides free online training courses on neurodiversity,
     which can be accessed here:
     https://exceptionalindividuals.com/candidates/online-workshops-training-uk/

4   The University of Derby provides free online courses on autism, Asperger's and
     ADHD. It can be accessed here:

     https://www.derby.ac.uk/short-courses-cpd/online/free-courses/understanding-
     autism-aspergers-and-adhd/

The ADHD Foundation provides a wealth of information for educators and their website
can be found here:
https://www.adhdfoundation.org.uk/

The British Dyslexia Association also has information for educators and their
weblink is here:
https://www.bdadyslexia.org.uk/

Chapter 15

Learning in non-assessed, virtual and alternate environments

Sarah Page, Gillian Ferguson, Kirsty Shanley and Ayana Horton Ifekoya

By the end of this chapter, you will be able to:

1 Describe learning opportunities in non-traditional practice settings.
2 Explore opportunities offered by virtual and simulated practice learning.
3 Identify practical approaches to negotiating and managing diverse practice placements.
4 Plan and evaluate arrangements for non-traditional practice learning arrangements.

Introduction

In this chapter, we will explore the diversity of practice learning settings with a focus on non-assessed, virtual and alternate environments. Building on earlier chapters, we will consider the essence and nature of practice learning in diverse types of placements. We will consider what constitutes an alternate environment, how to ensure that these meet the requirements of respective standards and equip learners for practice. Demand for relevant practice learning opportunities continues to increase across professions and workforce groups. Increased recruitment targets for the health and social care workforce have further exacerbated an already pinched sector (Kings Fund, 2022). This has led to creative developments across diverse health, social work, social care and third-sector (voluntary) services to enhance availability and expand opportunities. Ensuring that any practice learning meets the requirements of respective standards and effectively equips learners for practice needs to remain firmly at the heart of any alternative to traditional places and spaces for learning. The chapter explores the challenges and opportunities of facilitating learning and supporting learners within these settings.

Activity 1

Think about practice learning in the context of your role or responsibility. Reflect on what kinds of practice learning arrangements are required in this context.

- Where are learners traditionally placed for any formal practice learning?
- Who organised these placements and how are arrangements made?
- Identify any examples of unusual or non-traditional placements that you are aware of from your experience.
- What kinds of non-assessed placements happen in your setting?

DOI: 10.4324/9781003358602-15

Changes in roles and provision of services in health and social care have presented challenges and opportunities for students to expand their learning through practice in non-traditional, diverse and alternate practice learning environments. There is a responsibility for approved educational institutions, employer partners and professional regulatory bodies to prepare students for working in very different practice contexts once qualified' therefore, practice placement learning experiences must align to the current trends and expectations. This next section will discuss what we mean by non-traditional, diverse and alternate practice learning environments, their value and place in a student's professional education.

Non-traditional, diverse and alternate practice learning environments

Non-traditional practice learning environments might be those in emerging service areas where students have not always been placed. Recently, these have also been known as role-emerging or contemporary placements, those which reflect the changing trends and needs of services, adapting to new ways of working and using professional skills across boundaries. Creative developments in placement provision in health and social care span the last few decades, as a valuable way to nurture the skills of autonomous practice, to respond to the changing profile of workforce roles and meet increasing demands for learning opportunities. Non-traditional placements encourage students, and those supporting them, to develop their scope of practice in the context of health and social care. Students can critically develop their ideas, knowledge and skills, including being much more pragmatic and innovative. All learning through direct practice should generate and promote the development of professional identity, where students gain a stronger understanding of self and clarity about the workforce role.

Workplace settings that have not traditionally offered placements, or where there have been shifts in which students and apprentices undertake supervised learning are also in the scope of what we explore in this chapter. Non-traditional placements are often within environments where a specific profession has yet to be established and developed. Alternative and non-traditional placement arrangements have also stemmed from the changing partnerships and integrated service configurations that characterise current health and social care. Diverse practice learning environments are a key consideration for the sustainability of different professions as health and social care continues to expand into practice areas to support people experiencing intersecting issues in their lives. Services have also had to change to respond to changing demographic and socio-political trends. This includes the impact of issues such as poverty, homelessness, refugee and asylum seeker status. There are long-established and newer third-sector organisations with considerable expertise who are working increasingly in partnership with universal and specialist services to respond to health and social care needs. Many services have not previously considered supporting student placements or may have offered ad-hoc or shadowing opportunities. The most important factor is that any practice learning experience is meaningful and has benefit for both the student and the organisation in terms of shared learning.

In one example, occupational therapy (OT) student placements were traditionally arranged in hospitals, older people's care facilities and community health services. In more recent times, students can be placed in voluntary and independent sectors. This has led to broadening the scope, awareness and understanding of the OT role in different services, leading to a strengthening and appreciation of the profession. Alternate practice learning environments include those in the third sector, in charitable organisations, social enterprises and also in private services. These are termed 'alternate' only because they have not been part of original arrangements in professional or workforce training when educational programmes have been established in nursing, medicine, allied health professions, social care and social work. Alternate placements are sometimes also away from service settings, in research projects, professional organisations and in leadership, strategic or supporting teams. Placements across health and social care need to be rich in diversity, culture and inclusivity for people using the services, staff and learners within them. Considering where these rich spaces and places for learning are, can support creativity in thinking about blended placement arrangements where students can experience different forms of practice, transfer their skills and knowledge and promote understanding of different professional roles with colleagues.

There is no doubt that the context and delivery of health and social care services will continue to change. Crimlisk (2019) highlights the need for educational partnership models that support students to work across boundaries in response to the NHS Long Term Plan (NHS England, 2019). We will consider more details and examples of different types of placements in this chapter and the role of stakeholders in working together to expand the capacity of quality learning opportunities for the future.

Private, voluntary and independent sector placements

Where placements are arranged out of the NHS or a local authority, practice learning may be facilitated within a partnership or network of services. Individual services in the private, voluntary (or third sector) and independent services are often commissioned by NHS and aligned with priority areas of health and social care. The scope of services is very broad, ranging from personal or residential care to specialist services focusing on specific issues. There is no homogenous group of services, and it is essential to recognise the opportunities for learning where there are appropriate arrangements.

Third-sector (voluntary) services often have their origin in collective action against discrimination and there can be excellent learning opportunities for health and social care students to grapple with the underlying issues that lead to health, disease, inequality and social disadvantage. Many third-sector organisations also have extensive long-standing experiences of offering formal placements to students from many professions. One example is third-sector addiction services, which have historically offered a broad range of supervised nursing, social work, psychology, psychotherapy and counselling placements depending on their nature. In some innovative arrangements, nursing students have been encouraged to focus on a charity or issue of their interest to develop their learning (Thomas, 2022). The NHS Long Term Plan (NHS England, 2019) has proven to be a catalyst for change in how professional education reorientates to sector needs and shifting workforce roles. The scope of opportunities is vast; however, there are also challenges in developing effective practice learning placements across diverse and new arenas.

Learners can feel anxious about their practice learning experiences and particularly so when placed in a non-traditional context. There are numerous myths about employ-ability prospects and quality of practice learning amongst students that are perpetuated in organisations. It is important to recognise and appreciate different services, the significance of third-sector provision and expertise. Third-sector services represent some of the most creative and outcome-focused of services and many operate from an authentic co-production or people-powered approach. Beresford (2019) summarises the importance of co-produced knowledge, involvement and participation in health and social care. Practice learning provides an incredible opportunity for developing learning generated from experiential knowledge.

Irrespective of setting, any effective learning opportunity must recognise the learning needs, professional/workforce training standards and the specific requirements of any placement. One of the specific issues for third-sector placements is ensuring that the host agency has a sound knowledge of the professional area of the student or learner. There may or may not be members of staff who have appropriate qualifications to assess formal placements and arrangements must be negotiated clearly in advance for safe, ethical practice and for learners to have a fair opportunity to learn and be assessed. Doing the groundwork to establish clear and agreed-upon arrangements for any placements is vital, but this is true for any setting, something we will return to at the end of this chapter.

Activity 2

Reflect on the types of placements discussed so far in the chapter and identify any opportunities that there might be in your local area.

- What kind of placement opportunities are required in your area of practice?
- Where are services that match specialist areas of practice or roles?
- Are there any untapped placement opportunities in your own team or setting?
- How can partnership approaches help develop placement opportunities?

Placements within secure settings and the justice system

There is a wide range of secure settings and services within the justice system where students may gain valuable practice placement experiences. Students may have their practice placements in mental health or forensic units. Mental health hospitals may have secure units for individuals with severe mental illnesses who pose risks to themselves or others. Forensic hospitals are specialised medical facilities that provide treatment and care to people who have been involved in the criminal justice system and have mental health issues or psychiatric disorders. These facilities are designed to address the intersection of mental health and the legal system, particularly for individuals who have been found not guilty by reason of insanity, are deemed incompetent to stand trial or require psychiatric evaluation and treatment while incarcerated.

Students may also have placements in correctional facilities, such as prisons, jails, and detention centres. These are secure facilities designed to house people who have been convicted of crimes and sentenced to serve a period of incarceration as part of their punishment. This might include juvenile detention centres or halfway houses. Juvenile detention centres are facilities for minors who have committed delinquent acts and are awaiting adjudication or serving sentences. Halfway houses are transitional residences for individuals nearing the end of their sentences, intended to help them reintegrate into society gradually. There are also other types of secure care environments across different geographic areas for children and young people who are looked after away from home under statutory arrangements. Justice settings and services are configured differently and vary considerably across U.K. nations in terms of their underpinning policies, guidance, frameworks and related approaches to practice; therefore, an appreciation of your local context would be important in planning for practice learning.

Students working in secure settings and within the justice system experience unique learning opportunities due to the complex and often specialised nature of these settings. Secure settings can be volatile, providing students with valuable experience in crisis management and de-escalation techniques. Students also get invaluable experience navigating challenging workplace relationships, since patients in these facilities may exhibit challenging behaviours due to factors like incarceration stress, mental health issues or substance abuse. Working within the justice system exposes students to unique legal and ethical challenges, fostering a deep under-standing of these issues. Since students in these settings can be exposed to disturbing details of crimes, the duty of welfare to students is paramount to prevent vicarious trauma and a trauma-informed supervisory approach essential. Students who are learning in these settings often develop strong resilience and adaptability skills, which can be valuable in any healthcare setting. In addition, students in these settings can become advocates for improving healthcare and mental health services within the justice system, contributing to positive change. Lastly, working in these types of settings promotes understanding of the social determinants of health because these settings provide a unique and concentrated perspective on how various social factors can significantly impact the health and wellbeing of individuals involved in the criminal justice system.

These learning opportunities are not without challenges. There can be a stigma associated with working in the justice system, which may affect a student's willingness to take on such a placement. Working in secure settings, such as prisons or forensic hospitals, can be inherently risky due to the potential for violence or security breaches. Students must learn to prioritise safety while delivering care. Although this is at the fore of planning in secure settings, dynamic risk assessment is an important issue for all placement settings. Also, secure settings may have limited access to medical equipment, medications and technology. Students must adapt to these constraints while still providing effective care. In addition, students in these settings often face complex ethical dilemmas related to issues like patient confidentiality, involuntary treatment and the balance between security and patient care. Lastly, security measures and regulations can limit students' autonomy in decision-making and treatment planning, which can be frustrating.

Case study: Occupational therapy students in secure environments

The Brunel University, London, placements team placed a second-year MSc occupational therapy student at a high-security psychiatric facility located in the United Kingdom. The hospital is operated by the National Health Service (NHS) and is designed to house and treat individuals who have severe mental illness and pose a significant risk to themselves or others. A controlled and therapeutic environment is provided for patients who receive specialised care, therapy and support with a focus on their long-term recovery and public safety.

Occupational therapists at the hospital play a vital role in the multi-disciplinary treatment team, focusing on helping patients with severe mental illnesses develop the skills and strategies necessary to regain independence and improve their overall wellbeing. They assess patients' functional abilities and create individualised treatment plans aimed at enhancing their daily living skills, social interactions and vocational readiness. Occupational therapists may engage patients in various therapeutic activities and interventions, such as art therapy, vocational training and cognitive-behavioural techniques, to promote recovery, self-esteem and a sense of purpose. Their ultimate goal is to empower patients to reintegrate into the community successfully while ensuring they pose no harm to themselves or others, aligning with the hospital's mission of rehabilitation and risk management.

Although some students may be afraid to go on placements in secure settings, this particular student said she requested the placement because she wanted to work in this type of setting upon graduation. The student stated she really enjoyed the placement. She was initially on an assertive rehabilitation ward and then moved to a medium secure ward. As part of her orientation to the placement, she got training on how to set boundaries with patients, personality disorders, security and prevention/management of violence and aggression. A typical day for her was she would arrive and go through security, which she described as sort of like going through an airport. Then she would walk to the office and go over the plans for the day with her supervisor. Next, she and her supervisor would have a one to one or a group therapy session followed by a debrief on the session. After that, it would be lunch time. After lunch, they would have another therapy session, followed by another debrief. The student said the first few weeks were emotionally challenging because she was dealing with the guilt of feeling empathy for the patients, some of whom had done horrific things to others. She said she had to try not to let the patients' history influence their therapy by remembering that when they did their crimes they were unwell.

From the student's perspective, some of the benefits of having this type of placement was that she was able to develop her risk assessment skills and become more self-aware. Some of the challenges of this placement were that she could not go on the ward alone for safety reasons; everything required lots of planning, so everything took a long time, and dealing with residual emotions at the end of the day. To deal with these challenges she took advantage of the weekly reflective meetings offered by the psychology team. She also attempted to switch off after work by jogging and reading. She said that part of the reason she was able to adjust is she had a really supportive supervisor, but if she didn't it would have been really difficult. She recommended that future students on these types of placements got more support on how to deal with the harrowing aspects of patients' histories.

Activity 3

Reflect on what it might be like for a student to go on placement in a secure setting or within the justice system?

1   What reservations might you or your students have if you/they were allocated a placement in a secure setting or justice system? How would you allay those concerns?
2   What strategies would you use or advise your students to use to switch off at the end

of the day after being on a placement where you work with people who have committed crimes?

3   What attributes do you think a student needs to have to be successful on a placement in a secure setting or justice system?

Arm's-length supervision

Arm's-length, long-arm or indirect supervision are terms that have traditionally referred to a person who is supported by an off-site practice educator and an on-site supervisor. This is often an arrangement where new placements are under development or where there are non-traditional placements. In some circumstances, this is used because of the pressures on the workforce in the setting and the capacity of the team to provide practice educators. In long-arm arrangements, the practice educator is registered with their relevant professional body and may be employed by another organisation or education institution. The implementation of this model offers students opportunities to undertake innovative placements that can very well extend beyond the NHS and social care. Long-arm supervision can promote a diversity of vital skill sets across a variety of diverse cultural and situational backgrounds. Overall, students gain a very valuable opportunity to learn about the different techniques and approaches in supporting patients and clients, where a focus subtly shifts onto a picture of an individual strengths and preferences while moving away from an illness/deficit focused. This allows students to develop the autonomy and the ability to communicate at a much higher level of expertise with patients and clients across whole life span difficulties, and more importantly support patients and clients with mental health needs. It is essential to carefully negotiate roles and boundaries with all those involved so that the student/ learner and other parties are clear. This may seem complex at the outset, but planning carefully will reap benefits. All placements rely on effective working relationships and energy spent supporting the development of these; acknowledging different skills and experience is hugely beneficial.

Using simulation to enhance practice learning experiences

Over the last few decades, technology has continued to enhance and shift the ways that we learn and opportunities for doing so. In practice learning, there have been many debates about the role of technology, and about the use of simulation to develop practice skills across professions. This can take many forms and it is important to be clear about what is meant by simulation in the context of professional learning. In healthcare, there are also recognised standards for the use of simulation (INACSL, 2021), which reflect the expertise in this field. These standards underline the importance of all aspects of the design of simulated learning with clear outcomes in mind. During the COVID-19 pandemic in 2020, many educational programmes experienced a crisis in practice learning as placements were suspended, which affected the progression of many healthcare and social work students. Arrangements to pivot to online teaching methods were made at this time. This led to rhetoric about using simulation and virtual placements in some areas that were in fact delivering teaching content online rather than virtual or simulated practice experience. It is essential to be clear so that the right learning solutions are in place and recognised as part of the design of any programme where technology is used. Examples of creative use of simulation for practice skills training is a different entity to the completion of required practice learning days in live placements.

Activity 4

Reflect on your knowledge or experience of technology-enhanced learning in your service area:

- What kinds of virtual learning opportunities are employed? Are these effective?
- How has simulation been embedded in any professional learning that you are aware of?
- Where are opportunities for creative developments in virtual and simulated learning in your practice area?

Case study: Blended digital placements in primary care

A recent example has been the development of creative approaches in general practice (GP) within the east of England, where there are many challenges facing student placements, including time and estates capacity to host a student. This has led to opportunities for innovation and creativity to create exposure to this practice area and inspire the future workforce.

One of these opportunities involved the use of a blended digital placement for University of Bedfordshire nursing students, making use of developments in virtual learning, creating a robust combination of theory and practical learning. The digital placement consists of three days a week of virtual learning, completing a carefully mapped timetable of modules related to skills and knowledge specific to general practice nursing. This intersperses with opportunities to attend interactive webinars from expert speakers in their field. The learning modules consist of self-directed study, videos, quizzes and short tests. Each virtual day concludes with a group tutorial from experienced practice nurses that offers a chance to practice what has been learned such as consultation skills and ask questions to deepen knowledge. The student then has a unique opportunity to attend a placement in a GP surgery for two days a week. This offers the learner the chance to put the theory into practice in a safe environment with full supervision. In addition, each learner has a 1:1 with their virtual assessor three times over the placement to conduct the initial, middle and end-point interviews to discuss learning goals and actions.

Each practice placement was audited in order to ensure that the GP was a safe and conducive learning environment. This also facilitated collaborative working with the placement, the university and the primary care training hub. The learners are supported by a virtual assessor, virtual supervisor and practice supervisor and have the added support of legacy nurses who can visit whilst on their placement.

Evaluation of the placement was positive and encouraging, with learners scoring their placement experience as 4.8/5 for extremely satisfied. There is a scope for this to be a viable option for other branches of nursing, such as children and young people, mental health and learning disabilities as GP settings see patients from 'cradle to grave'. This placement could also be extended for paramedic science, physiotherapy and midwifery students who are becoming more embedded within GP settings.

Negotiating, managing and evaluating practice learning opportunities

Some of the challenges for people arranging placements in non-traditional settings include that students may be supervised by someone who is not in their specific discipline. There may also be generic roles that don't allow the student to develop their professional identity. There are, however, many assumptions about what learning is possible and there are numerous benefits of diverse placement opportunities to students that are outlined in this chapter. In summary, these benefits include:

- Promotes understanding of the expertise and services offered in diverse settings
- Development of autonomous practitioner skills
- Increases pool of placements in multi-agency context
- Students are forced to consider the wider applicability of concepts and theories learned than they would in more traditional settings
- Opportunity for students to advocate and promote their professional skills
- Fosters practice placements relevant to changing work practices and roles

In essence, there are always things to consider in any setting. Careful plans are therefore important for any practice learning placements to be successful. It can be helpful to have a clear reminder of things to check to make sure everything is in place. Services and people coordinating placements are increasingly under pressure, but planning carefully can promote a strong learning community that has wide-reaching benefits. Table 15.1 presents a set of criteria to check that the necessary arrangements for placements are set up, reviewed and evaluated to feed into future planning.

Table 15.1 Criteria for placement development

Negotiating	✓
Are the requirements of the student understood in the prospective placement setting?	
How would the placement need to be adapted to meet the learning/learner requirements?	
Where is the specific professional expertise, supervision and guidance going to come from? Is this available or are other arrangements being made to support this? Are the roles of different people clear?	
Does the potential placement have the necessary resources to support the student?	
Managing	
How will the arrangements be monitored? Are there additional measures for ensuring the relevant range of work tasks and learning opportunities are in place?	
Are there additional opportunities needed for the student?	
Is additional support or expertise required for the placement setting?	
Are there opportunities for the student to share learning with peers during the placement to promote understanding of the broader professional context?	

(Continued)

Table 15.1 (Continued)

Evaluating	
Have students had a robust learning opportunity and been fairly assessed?	
How will you gather feedback during and after the placement and who needs to provide this?	
How will you collaboratively review the arrangements with the agency, educational establishment and key stakeholders?	
How will you feed information into a clear review cycle for improving next steps?	
Additional things to check/notes	

Activity 5

Explore the components of the checklist in Table 15.1, for negotiating, managing and evaluating practice learning in diverse practice learning settings:

- Identify three questions that you think are most important. Why do you think these are important?
- Is there anything you would add to the checklist?
- How would you use the checklist to guide the development of placements in your setting?

Conclusion

This chapter has explored some of the ways in which practice learning placements are continuing to evolve in health and social care across diverse environments. Creative approaches can increase the range of placements offered and the spectrum of skills and knowledge of students in different professions. Care, however, needs taken in planning, managing and reviewing placements in any settings to support effective relationships and arrangements that offer robust opportunities for students to learn.

References

Beresford, P (2019) 'Public participation in health and social care: Exploring the co-production of knowledge', *Frontiers of Sociology*, 3, p. 41.

Crimlisk, H (2019) *Educational partnerships with the third sector*. The Health Foundation. Available at https://www.health.org.uk/news-and-comment/blogs/educational-partnerships-with-the-third-sector-a-model-to-address-nhs (accessed 17 July 2023).

INACSL Standards Committee, Hallmark, B, Brown, M, Peterson, DT, Fey, M, Morse, C (2021, September) 'Healthcare simulation standards of best practice TM professional development', *Clinical Simulation in Nursing*, 58, pp. 5–8.

Kings Fund (2022) *NHS workforce: Our position*. Available at https://www.kingsfund.org.uk/projects/positions/nhs-workforce (accessed 17 July 2023).

NHS England (2019) *NHS long term plan NHS England*. Available at https://www.longtermplan.nhs.uk/wp-content/uploads/2019/08/nhs-long-term-plan-version-1.2.pdf (accessed 17 July 2023).

Thomas, A (2022) 'Encouraging collaboration between student nurses and the third sector', *Nursing Times* [online], 118, p. 12.

Chapter 16

Transitioning to the role of practice assessor/educator and beyond

Mark Wareing and Meriel Norris

By the end of this chapter, you will be able to:

1 Differentiate supervision and assessment of practice.
2 Identify the challenges and opportunities of dual supervision and assessment roles.
3 Analyse leadership in the context of supporting learners and creating new practice education experiences.
4 Evaluate the range of career development opportunities open to the aspirant educator.

Introduction

In this final chapter, we will return to the practice of the supervisor, assessor and practice educator in comparison to other roles that are required for students and apprentices to be supported and assessed in practice. Allied health professions and social work students within the United Kingdom are currently supported by practice educators who have a dual role in supporting and assessing students, in contrast to nursing, midwifery and operating department practitioner students who have designated assessors that conduct final/summative assessment. The challenges of fulfilling both roles will be examined in addition to a consideration of the qualities needed to be a confident assessor of students and apprentices. This also includes a consideration of supervision at an advanced level of practice, where we consider the case study of Sanjay.

In the section on leadership, we progress our journey, considering where a focus on practice could lead you professionally. We will explore models and styles of leadership prior to an examination of two case studies, featuring Tanya and Tom, who were able to demonstrate their leadership skills in order to create new practice education experiences for pre- and post-registration students through co-production, which enhanced learning for all. Lastly, the chapter will conclude with a survey of career opportunities available for experienced practice educators, supervisors and assessors and strategies for transitioning into an academic role including managing time and workstreams.

Revisiting assessor and educator role descriptors

Activity 5 in Chapter 1 required you to identify whether you had a supporting or assessing role, what training and preparation was required, what type of learners you were permitted to support and other colleagues you would need to work with as an educator.

DOI: 10.4324/9781003358602-16

Activity 1

1 Access the relevant Professional Standard Regulatory Body (PSRB) guidance for practice learning and identify your role in supporting students and apprentices within your clinical and therapeutic area.

2 Complete Table 16.1 in order to make sense of staff responsibilities.

You will see that the first row has already been completed.

3. If you have answered 'don't know' to any of the questions, be sure to arrange a meeting with someone in your workplace who can help you identify the correct answer; this could be a more experienced practice supervisor, assessor or educator; a clinical learning facilitator; learning environment lead or link lecturer/tutor from your local university.

Table 16.1 Making sense of staff responsibilities for students and apprentices

Activity questions:	In my allocated practice role: (e.g. Practice Educator, Practice Supervisor, Practice Assessor)	Other allocated practice role: (e.g. if support and assessment roles are separate)
Can I complete a learning agreement or write learning outcomes with a student/apprentice? If not, who can?	Yes, because I am a practice supervisor	Practice assessors can also do this
Can I fulfil indirect or arm's-length supervision? If not, who can?		
Can I assess that a student or apprentice is competent or proficient? If not, who can?		
Can I provide feedback to inform formative and summative assessment?		
Can I complete a formative (mid-point) assessment?		
Can I raise a concern regarding a student or complete a danger of fail report? If not, who can?		
Can I write an action plan if concerned about a student or apprentice's performance? If not, who can?		
Can I complete a summative/final assessment? If not, who can?		
Can I confirm a student or apprentice's progression or complete a statement to that effect? If not, who can?		

Challenges of being a supervisor and assessor

Providing direct support as well as assessing the same student has been known to present challenges, particularly when a strong bond has been created between the learner and the educator (Brown *et al.*, 2020) who has the dual responsibility for supervision and conducting summative assessments (Baluyot and Blomberg, 2019; Helminen *et al.*, 2016). Professional bodies in the United Kingdom, such as the Nursing and Midwifery Council (NMC) and College of Operating Department Practitioners (CODP), separated the two roles previously fulfilled by mentors (NMC, 2023; CODP, 2021), in an attempt to counter failure-to-fail situations and ensure that practice assessment decisions were informed by a range of sources of feedback. The purpose of Activity 1 was to assist you to identify your role in the support of students, whilst acknowledging that practice supervisors play a key role in preparing students for assessment. Practice educators and practice assessors can make open, fair and transparent assessment decisions more confidently when evidence is drawn from practice staff, patients, clients and service users that confirms the final decision, as we saw in Chapter 14. In Chapters 5 and 6, it was argued that it is critical for assessment evidence to be fully documented, enabling the practice educator/assessor to be held accountable for their assessment decisions.

Making the decision to transition from being a practice supervisor to an assessor and preparing to conduct your first summative assessment is a significant responsibility given the implications of a summative assessment on the student and apprentice and the consequences if a learner successfully appeals against an assessment decision. Failing an underperforming student can be a challenging and difficult experience and it is acknowledged that the separation of support and assessment roles may not entirely eradicate the likelihood of a student not failing when they should have been.

Hunt's (2019) study attempted to identify the key personal characteristics of assessors who were prepared to fail underperforming students. These were:

Solidarity: Research participants interviewed in the study emphasised their professional role in maintaining public trust and ensuring that patients received high-quality care. Not only did they possess a strong sense of loyalty to the standards of their profession, but were determined to uphold professional values based on an interconnectedness with colleagues and a commitment to being a gatekeeper for their profession.

Tenacity: Failing the student was described as a difficult process, as there were a number of challenges and obstacles encountered when supporting and assessing an underperforming student, which required persistent determination.

Audacity: Research participants reported having a set of qualities that together signified audaciousness by challenging convention and not giving in to intimidation from students. Additionally, participants described being ready to challenge learners at later stages of the process, as further evidence came to light.

Integrity: Participants presented themselves as being consistent in their decision-making, which was based on their strongly held moral principles.

Dependability: During times of tension, participants needed composure and commitment to see the process through and meet their obligations by communicating their intention with clarity.

The characteristics described in the above study are a reminder that undertaking assessment (as a practice educator) or transitioning to the role of a practice assessor, following appropriate experience as a practice supervisor, is a significant responsibility. Line managers, heads of department, team and ward managers and learning environment leads need to work collaboratively to ensure that registered health and social work professionals are selected carefully for the role of an assessing practice educator or practice assessor, whilst valuing the role that practice supervisors play in contributing to mid-point review meetings and preparing students and apprentices for summative assessments.

Activity 2

Hunt (2019, p. 1482) argued that the key attributes of assessors (solidarity, tenacity, audacity, integrity, dependability) form a 'core of steel' that should prevent students and apprentices from being registered with a professional standard regulatory body 'when they should not be there':

1 What, if any, 'enablers' exist within your workplace area that would support you to become an assessor that had a 'core of steel'?
2 What, if any, 'barriers' exist within your workplace area that would prevent you from practising as an assessor with a 'core of steel'?

Table 16.2 presents a self- assessment tool to assist line managers, heads of department, team and ward managers and learning environment leads to select suitable registered practitioners to become assessors. The tool comprises of five 'continuums' that can be used to assess a potential assessor's tendency towards one or other of the two opposing characteristics. Hunt (2019) argued that identification with the qualities towards the left of each continuum indicated a close alignment with the 'core of steel' needed to be an effective assessor, whilst identifying with the contrasting characteristics suggested the person would not be well aligned to the assessor role. The table has been adapted to suggest a range of developmental strategies to become an effective practice assessor that might overcome the 'barriers' identified in the previous activity.

Table 16.2 Assessing with a core of steel: self-assessment tool

Assessor ready if …	Continuum	Development required if …	Suggested developmental actions
Solid Loyal to professional standards allegiance to patients, clients, service users	⬄	Yielding Malleable and pliant Gives way under pressure	• Clinical supervision • Personal development coaching • Assertiveness training • Coaching around operationalisation of professional practice education standards and assessment documentation
Tenacious Will not relinquish principles Prepared to fight to fail	⬄	Tentative Guarded and hesitant Unsettled by change	• Practice assessor/educator refresher session • Shadowing of an experienced Assessor • Third-party support from university link lecturer/tutor • Personal development around managing change and observation of effective change practitioners

(Continued)

Table 16.2 (Continued)

Assessor ready if ...	Continuum	Development required if ...	Suggested developmental actions
Audacious Bold, courageous and assertive Undaunted when threatened		Reticent Cautious in speaking out Reserved and deferential	• Assertiveness training • Observation of an effective communicator, practitioners, leaders • Engagement in values-based reflection • Buddy-buddy with experienced assessor
Integrity Works to clear principles Focused on what is right	⟺	Nonchalant Casual and informal Carefree approach	• Root cause analysis activity to uncover personal stance • Support to engage in appreciative inquiry • Adoption of an ethical deliberative framework to develop ethical competence e.g. seeing/perception, knowing, reflection, doing, being (Gallagher, 2006)
Dependable Follow process consistently Resilient and would do it again	⟺	Changeable Adjustable and varying Sporadically committed	• Direct support from practice education team, practice education facilitator, university link lecturer/ tutor during formative and summative assessment • Contextualisation of proficiencies and/or competencies to own practice area, clinical speciality and local expected standards of work

Source: Adapted from Hunt (2019, p. 1483).

Preparing for supervisor, assessor and practice educator training

This book has been written with a range of readers in mind, including final-year health and social work students who may be exploring practice learning perhaps for the first time and registered professionals preparing to undertake supervisor, assessor and educator training normally after a period of post-registration experience and training called preceptorship.

Activity 3

This next activity aims to assist in identifying the supervisor, assessor and educator training appropriate to your current employment within a health and social work setting:

1   If you have not already done so, arrange an annual appraisal or individual personal development review (IPR) meeting with your line manager to agree what educational role is required for your team, department, ward or practice area in

the context of the trainees, learners, students or apprentices needing support with their practice education.

2   In preparation for the above meeting, contact your employing organisations' education and training department to identify the range of supervisor, assessor and educator training on offer and for whom.

3   Undertake an internet search for relevant professional organisations that provide open access preparatory resources to help you prepare for your formal supervisor, assessor or educator training and provide ongoing support and continuous professional development. See 'helpful resources' at the end of this chapter.

Supervising in advanced practice roles

Up until now we have considered the role of the supervisor, assessor or educator and the skills required in multiple different settings. Much of this has been focused on pre-registration students and apprentices who will join an established team for the period of their practice-based learning. The learners are often unknown to the supervisor or assessor prior to the period of learning and the setting is frequently new to the learner.

However, learning and supervision is an ongoing process for all health and social work professionals and increasing emphasis is placed on advancing practice through focused work-based learning. This is evidenced in the requirement for work-based learning in training for recognised roles such as the advanced clinical practitioner (HEE 2017), or specific advanced skills such as non-medical prescribing and injection therapy amongst several others. Furthermore, as practitioners become more experienced, it is expected that they also influence transformational improvements within healthcare services, which includes educational culture, not just of individuals but also their teams and indeed the culture of the organisation in which they are employed (HEE 2017). These requirements create a series of new opportunities for senior practice staff but also dilemmas and the need for further skill development. We will explore some of these through case studies featuring Tanya and Tom. The purpose is not to give solutions as all the approaches and techniques in the previous chapters can be drawn upon. Rather, it is to explore additional considerations when supervising in this advanced context or indeed learning how to influence education and develop leadership skills within the workplace.

Case study 1: Supervising and being supervised by team members from different professional backgrounds

As noted above, supervision in the specialist setting is frequently done by colleagues with whom there may be ongoing relations and history. They may also be completed by team members from different specialities in which expectations and professional scope of practice may vary. In the following example, we explore some of these issues:

Sanjay is a specialist neuro occupational therapist (OT) who works on the stroke unit in a large teaching hospital. He is undertaking an MSc in advanced clinical practice in which observation of him implementing his knowledge and skills is a regular part of his supervision and embedded in his assessments. As the most senior OT in the hospital in this speciality, Sanjay is being supervised by Kathy, a physiotherapist who has been employed as an advanced practitioner for five years. The pair have worked together for six years and have collaborated on many development projects in recent years.

On a recent observation, Kathy has noted that Sanjay could broaden his focus of assessment to consider other body systems, such as cardiovascular capacity, when working on functional activities and could do more to explain this adequately to the patients. While she was not concerned with safety in this instance, she felt that this additional assessment was key to a comprehensive risk assessment. She was aware that this assessment of cardiovascular capacity may not be routine in occupational therapy training and practice, but was relevant for advanced practice in the context of stroke rehabilitation. They are due a supervision session, where Kathy will share her observation. This is the first time she will be raising direct concerns with his practice.

Sanjay felt the session itself had gone well, but is aware that he has struggled a little to work beyond his normal boundaries of OT practice clinically. He knows Kathy well and has sensed a slight change in her behaviour towards him since the session. He is nervous about the supervision meeting.

Activity 4

Thinking about the forthcoming supervision session, consider the following questions:

1   What approach could Kathy take to introduce and discuss the issue raised effectively?
2   How may the different professional backgrounds and experience levels impact this discussion and how can that be duly acknowledged?
3   How can Kathy support Sanjay in developing confidence in his wider scope of practice?
4   How may their previous relationship impact on this supervisory conversation and what steps could be taken to consider this?

It is important to remember that the completion of supervisor, assessor and educator training may lead to the support of post-registration students such as Sanjay and learners undertaking more specialised programmes of study, such as non-medical prescribing (NMP).

Leadership

Throughout this book we have explored a range of key features within the landscape of practice that are dependent on the role of practice educators, supervisors and assessors such as the enhancement of learning environments; assessing practice and performance; facilitating learning conversations 'that matter' and supporting the health and wellbeing of students and apprentices whilst meeting the requirements of professional standard regulatory body guidance. Given the requirement of educators, assessors and supervisors to be a role model, it is important that leadership skills are developed and demonstrated; not least as learning takes place at a time when meeting the needs of clients and patients is essential. In this section, we will explore a range of leadership styles and approaches to assist educators in balancing their roles as supervisors, assessors and practitioners.

Barr and Dowding (2012, p. 11) argue that 'leadership is both an art and a science. An art because of the many skills and qualities that cannot be learned via a textbook but a science because of the growing body of knowledge that describes the leadership process, leadership skills and the application of these elements within a given practice area'. Contemporary health and social work practices operate as an art and science within a landscape of practice where informal learning is necessary for the acquisition of leadership skills within practice settings.

Activity 5

Think about your line manager, head of department or team leader:

1   What positive effect does this person have on the behaviour of their staff?
2   What strategies do they use to ensure that the department, team or ward provides a safe and effective service?
3   To what extent have you modelled your own leadership style on this person?
4   What leadership skills do you most admire in this person?
5   In what areas would you say the person is less effective?

It is beyond the scope of this chapter to present a comprehensive exploration of leadership within practice learning settings. Being familiar with the range of leadership models and identifying situations where they might be applicable is useful in determining which leadership style is appropriate when balancing your role as a clinician, practitioner and educator within a given practice setting. Table 16.3 presents seven common leadership models ranging from the 'qualities' or 'trait's' approach where leadership is regarded as an innate ability, through to a model that views the role of a leader within purely ethical terms.

The 'qualities or traits' model of leadership is sometimes referred to as the 'great person theory' or 'great man of history' model, although attempts to identify the particular characteristics of leaders is highly subjective, particularly when their traits are reflective of their individualism. The model can also be criticised as it fails to consider the effect of situational factors and may privilege those who possess characteristics linked to their social background or education. The 'functional or group' model assumes leadership can be learnt, although organisations would not be able to remain successful if they simply waited for leaders to come along. A strength of the model is its suggestion that there is a relationship between management and leadership. The behavioural model links to Activity 3, as the approach suggests that leaders are required to establish trust, respect and rapport using two-way communication, where the leader defines group interaction. However, the model seems to ignore the influence of the organisational culture, which may undermine a leader despite their communication abilities. The 'situational/contingency' model would seem particularly relevant to volatile, uncertain, changing, ambiguous and super-complex practice settings, but is dependent on people possessing appropriate knowledge and skills within a given situation regardless of their effectiveness as a leader. One further criticism of the model lies in the requirement for practitioners to demonstrate accountability for their decisions, actions and omissions within settings where the use of evidence-based approaches is of particular importance. The transformational and inspirational models are perhaps the most attractive models for

Table 16.3 Models of leadership

Model of leadership	Characteristics 'in a nutshell'
Qualities or traits approach	Assumes leaders are born and not made. Leadership consists of certain inherited characteristics or personality traits. Focuses attention on the person in the job and not on the job itself.
Functional or group approach	Attention is faced on the functions and responsibilities of leadership, what the leader actually does and the nature of the group. Assumes leadership skills can be learned and developed.
Behavioural approach	The kinds of behaviour of people in leadership positions and the influence of group performance. Draws attention to range of possible managerial behaviour and importance of leadership style.
Situational/contingency approach	The importance of the situation. Interactions between variables involved in the leadership situation and patterns of behaviour. Belief that there is no single style of leadership appropriate to all situations.
Transformational approach	A process of engendering motivation and commitment, creating a vision for transforming the performance of the organisation and appealing to the higher ideals and values of followers.
Inspirational approach	Based on the personal qualities or charisma of the leader and the manner in which the leadership influence is exercised.
Servant approach	More a philosophy based on an ethical responsibility of leaders. A spiritual understanding of people and empowering people through honesty, respect, nurturing and trust.

Source: Adapted from Mullins (2004).

the promotion of learning and the influence of the educator on the student and apprentice, but could be regarded as being rather idealistic and may not be suitable for those whose thinking is more lateral than creative or transactional. Finally, the 'servant model' speaks to the moral virtuosity of health and social work practice and education, but could be criticised for its therapeutic emphasis and risks, creating a dependency culture that may pose a threat to the objectivity that is necessary within professional working relationships (Mullins, 2004).

At best it would seem that leadership models offer a somewhat limited explanatory framework in which to categorise general approaches to leadership roles that are primarily related to particular practice contexts, situations and specific service sectors. Given the complexity of the landscape of practice, a consideration of leadership styles places greater emphasis on the communicative action that characterises educational leadership.

Leadership styles

The Chartered Institute of Personnel and Development (CIPD, 2023) defines leadership as the process of understanding people's motivation and leveraging them to achieve a common goal comprising of three essential elements:

Self: Leaders must have self-awareness and effectively express their personal qualities.

Other people: Leaders must influence, motivate and inspire their stakeholders.

The job: Leaders should define, clarify and revise tasks that need to be achieved.

A leadership model needs to be translated into practice through the adoption of a leadership style in order for people to be prepared to follow their leader within a range of circumstances. Leaders may adopt a style that at times may be regarded as coercive, where the right balance of sanction, reward and direction is required. Such an approach may be necessary when supporting a student or apprentice to understand the consequences of poor participatory learning and inadequate preparation for practice assessments. An authoritative leadership style could be characterised as a leader who presents a clear vision and a long-term direction whilst demonstrating an ability to justify their actions. Such a leadership style might be appropriate when inducting a group of students or apprentices at the start of a substantial or lengthy practice education experience, or where the learner is expected to negotiate their own learning experiences in response to supervision that is 'long arm' or indirect. An affiliative learning style might be adopted in order to avoid conflict through the creation of a deep harmony between the learner and supervisor, perhaps when a student or apprentice has experienced a particularly traumatic practice experience or has been struggling with challenging situations outside of the placement area that are beyond their control. When students and apprentices are engaging in a peer-assisted learning experience supported by a coach, a democratic consensus-based leadership style may be deemed appropriate in addition to the leader engaging in 'pacesetting' to ensure that learning objectives are accomplished to a high level of excellence (Barr and Dowding, 2012, p. 17) whilst providing coaching to encourage the development of all learners.

Career development

In this next section, we will explore how practice supervisor, assessor and educator experience can be used as the basis of career development. There are a wide range of opportunities within health and social work for experienced supervisors, assessors and educators to progress to roles within social work, nursing, allied health professions, nursing and midwifery practice education teams, as learning facilitators, practice education facilitators and learning environment leads. Additionally, roles such as education and training leads and managers are open to experienced educators within local authorities, statutory services and large private, voluntary and independent organisations.

The next activity seeks to demystify the roles of academic staff within approved education institutes by highlighting the diversity of practice and professional experience that staff in learning and teaching roles possess.

Activity 6

Undertake an internet search of the profiles of academic staff who have responsibility for the delivery of pre-registration health and social work courses:

1 Select the staff profiles on the website of a college, faculty, school or department section of an approved education institution or university. Alternatively, you can

browse individual health and social work profession profiles via LinkedIn: https://gb. linkedin.com/

2   Explore the range of professional practice backgrounds that academic staff had prior to entering higher education.

3   Visit the job vacancy section of the website or browse job vacancies at the following websites:

- jobs.ac.uk
- Times Higher Educational Supplement (THES) [https://www.timeshighereducation. com/unijobs/]

4   Explore lecturer, tutor or teaching fellow posts most relevant to your own professional background. Education, teaching and lecturing posts can also be found on the Council of Deans of Health website: https://www.councilofdeans.org.uk/jobs/

Hopefully, the last activity will have highlighted the common entry requirements for practice staff considering a career within a formal educational establishment as well as the diversity of skills, experience and practice and professional and clinical interests that attract practice staff to learning, teaching, simulation and research roles.

In the next section, we will see how educational roles can be used as a springboard for the enhancement of practice education, the learning environment and improving outcomes for service users.

Case study 2: Expanding supervision and influencing broader educational practice

In this case study, we will explore the route Tanya took to expanding her career goals as a practice educator:

Tanya has been working as a pelvic health physiotherapist for 17 years and supports the development of the staff in her team through regular supervision. She is passionate about developing her local services but also expanding training in this field to students and newly qualified physiotherapy staff. Currently, students rarely come on placement in this specialist area and the trust does not employ band 5 staff in pelvic health. Consequently, recruiting specialised staff for available positions has become a challenge due to the limited educational opportunities.

As a first step, Tanya contacted a local university that has a large physiotherapy undergraduate programme. She was aware that they provided some minimal education in pelvic health to undergraduates and saw an opportunity to collaborate. Together with the university team, Tanya developed hybrid placements. These placements provided students with clinical experience, aligning with the part-time pelvic health team, as well as structured quality improvement projects related to the clinical area. Tanya's team presented workplace challenges for students to investigate, with support from university educators on non-clinical days. The placement also included specific days of clinical practice, complemented by more in-depth education both at the university and through structured work-based observations. In order to ensure both safety of patients but also support and development learning for the placement students, Tanya worked closely with the university team to understand the student's level of knowledge and devised a progressive plan to move from theory to practice over the six-week period. The first pilot version of the placement was evaluated by both staff and students, leading to valuable recommendations for future iterations.

Following her interactions with the university, she extended her connections and offered some time as a clinical lecturer. This both expanded the resources the university had to introduce students to the specialist area but also exposed Tanya to concepts such as curriculum design, evidence-based educational practices such as the flipped classroom and robust evaluation of her teaching. Over time, her confidence in her university teaching improved but also her practices within her clinical environment. Tanya revamped her in-service training sessions, identifying needs prior to planning sessions and always gathered anonymised feedback not just on content and her style but also what her staff members had gained.

This case study demonstrates Tanya's passion for pelvic health and how she enabled students to seek out opportunities to undertake a pelvic health placement. Over time, Tanya cemented her connection with the university through a permanent part-time teaching contract, while maintaining her clinical role. She successfully completed a postgraduate certificate in education and is currently using skills gained to create an educational development plan for a band 5 rotation role in her department.

Activity 7

Tanya utilised existing and new educational pathways to expand her own personal development, diversify her skills in work-based supervision and learning and to create new educational pathways to support specific service needs and design. Thinking about your specific context, consider the following questions:

1   How has your continuous professional development as a supervisor, assessor or educator been supported in practice?
2   Which areas do you have a particular interest in developing and where could you seek opportunities?
3   How could diversifying your supervisory/educational role support your service needs?
4   What are the first steps you could take to start this process?

Case study 3: Co-production as an opportunity to learn and develop skills and services

In their ambition to transform and improve services, advanced practitioners are expected to draw on expertise from many sources. Service users, also known as 'experts by experience', as well as stakeholders from other services, become invaluable in this endeavour. In the final case study, we are introduced to Tom, who utilised co-production to create a new approach to practice education experience whilst enhancing a clinical service:

Tom works within the musculoskeletal service in a diverse urban community setting and frequently supervises students. He and a final-year student whom he supervised recently conducted an audit exploring outcomes from the physiotherapy clinic based on multiple factors. The findings were complex but the data demonstrated a high rate of patients with diabetes seeking musculoskeletal services, but that successful outcomes were lower than in those without diabetes and particularly in-service users from racialised minority groups.

Following a discussion with his managers, Tom undertook a series of open meetings with different stakeholders. This included staff from the local diabetes centre, who frequently referred their clients to the musculoskeletal service. With their support, he also consulted with service users with diabetes who had been referred to his service. He and the wider team were careful to ensure there was appropriate representation in that group to hear from different demographic groups. He included his next student in these meetings, giving them specific roles such as 'meet and greet', minute talking and discussing the findings. These discussions resulted in some key insights.

These included;

- *The staff in the diabetes clinic are not fully aware of what services the musculo-skeletal team offers, when it is the most appropriate time to refer and what information the musculoskeletal team needs to assist in their screening and prioritisation process.*
- *The musculoskeletal team had knowledge gaps in the pathology of diabetes and its subsequent links with musculoskeletal problems and recovery processes.*
- *The service users were used to the diabetes clinic and managed their routine appointments into their everyday life. The musculoskeletal appointments were in a different venue unknown to them and on different dates and times. This combination created challenges for them in relation to work and life management. Many were not very clear why they had been referred to this team in the first place.*
- *Some service users associated the musculoskeletal service with simple exercise sheets, which they felt they could download from the internet. Others, who had attended their musculoskeletal appointment, felt that the team had focused on a single body part and not really considered that they had other complications related to their diabetes.*

Following this, Tom coordinated with the team to enact a number of changes. A series of cross-clinic/disciplinary education sessions were organised with content from the discussions and further detailed input from the respective teams. A leaflet was co-created with staff members from both clinical teams and service users to outline what the musculoskeletal service offered and some myth-busting statements in accessible lan-guage. Tom's student specifically supported this work as they had some skills in IT but also to support their own development of lay and professional language. A member of the musculoskeletal team arranged to spend one day a week situated in the diabetes clinic to support interaction and early-referral discussions. This resulted in a change in the referral guidelines used between the two teams.

Initial indications are that this collaboration has not only improved education across the teams, but also streamlined working practices and improved earlier uptake from service users. The two students involved gained valuable skills in clinical audit, collaborative working practices and effective communication while also having their own skills acknowledged.

Activity 8

In the light of the above case study, think about your practice and consider the following:

1   What other service or clinical areas do your services interact with (whether directly or indirectly)?
2   How much do you know about those services and how much do they know about yours?
3   How does your service area involve service users in educating the team about their perceptions and needs in service provision?
4   How can students who are on practice placements with you contribute to activities such as this?

Transitioning to an approved education institute

We saw in the case study featuring Tanya that it is possible to balance an academic and clinical role that some practitioners regard as essential in maintaining their clinical or professional credibility. You may have identified some lecturer-practitioner or 50:50 roles whilst undertaking Activity 6. An alternative opportunity is to contact your local approved educational institute or university to enquire into visiting lecturer or specialist lecturer roles, where you can secure a short-term paid contract to undertake hourly teaching or clinical assessment work to gain experience in working within the higher education sector.

Making the transition from professional or clinical practice to higher education can present a range of opportunities as well as challenges, particularly if you have gained significant experience and expertise in a role for a period of time and have become well established. Table 16.4 attempts to differentiate education environments from professional and clinical settings. Transitioning from a clinical/professional practitioner to an academic role can be challenging for newcomers as they move from a highly structured and client-needs orientated environment where their role might be 'reactive', to the academic setting, where there is flexibility around being on campus to teach, hold tutorials and attend face-to-face meetings. Whilst some learning and teaching is still provided online, the predominant structure within the university setting is around the delivery of formal teaching and simulated learning sessions based on a timetable (typically of 10–11 weeks) that ensures that a block or module of study is delivered with a blend of face-to-face, synchronous, asynchronous learning, seminars and tutorials in addition to students being assessed formatively and summatively by the end of the module.

Table 16.4 suggests that academic staff need to plan their diary in a prospective manner to ensure that taught sessions are delivered, students' work is assessed and moderated and module results are ready for examination progression and awarding boards; where students are identified who can progress to the next stage of their studies or when academic qualifications are awarded.

Table 16.4 Contrasting working environments

Characteristics	Educational	Practice/clinical
Organisation of work	Structured around timetabling, assessment, marking, tutorials, practicum, simulation and meetings; largely planned, orientated to term, semester, academic year to meet professional standard regulatory body/Ofsted approval requirements	Structured around meeting the immediate needs of patients, clients, families, service users; planned and unplanned; orientated to treatment sequelae, recovery or management models
Clientele	Students, apprentices, practice partners, professional standard regulatory bodies, Ofsted, other accrediting bodies, research funders	Patients, children, young people, families, service users, suppliers, service commissioners, statutory local authorities; other health and social work professionals within primary and secondary care
Nature of service	Higher education	Health and social work
Nature of productivity	Academic progression and graduate outcomes, attainment, civic engagement, industry partnerships, research, collaborative work, related to league tables (national and international)	Service provision, social justice, public health, related to care quality commission (CQC) outcomes
Resources	Student fees, research grants, income from business, intellectual property	Tax payer (via national insurance); patient/client as customer purchasing own services, therapy, treatment, diagnostic or surgical interventions
Use of IT	Business, finance, management, virtual and simulated learning, library and online learning	Data management, retrieval, electronic patient/client records, virtual healthcare, biochemical, diagnostic
Support services	Professional, administrative and technical	Clinical and administrative
Role of research	Knowledge generation, scholarly activity, income/grants, doctoral, Research Excellence Framework (REF)	Evidence-based medicine, healthcare practice, service evaluation, public health, service commissioning
Organisational culture	Related to academic category and standing of institution e.g. Russell Group, 'plate glass', technical, post-1992, Million Group	Related to quality standard outcomes and performance arising from CQC, safe-guarding, local authority funding
Public expectations	Generate next generation of professionals, research, innovation, science, development, technology, arts, civic engagement	Health, wellbeing, public health, disease and poverty eradication, social justice, fairness, community engagement

(Continued)

Table 16.4 (Continued)

Characteristics	Educational	Practice/clinical
Private expectations	Competition, income generation, academic standing nationally and internationally	Financial, corporate, clinical and integrated governance, competitive clinical/client outcomes, service commissioning
Communitarian expectations	Civic engagement, social mission, widening participation in education, inclusivity; addressing societies big/wicked problems	Accountable, accessible, funded services that meet the need of the individuals, groups, communities, region; addressing poverty, the disadvantaged, marginalised and vulnerable
Work-life balance	Balancing learning, teaching, research, scholarly activity, administration, pastoral support of students, apprentices; supporting learners in practice and simulated learning within a distinct course, programme/academic team; flexible/hybrid working commonplace	Requirement to provide 24-hour, seven-day week urgent and unplanned care utilising shift-work, on-call and rapid response for many clinical roles; significant service demands within post-pandemic environment that has led to waiting times and safe-guarding and mental health service demands and changes to delivery of health and social work intervention and services via online and hybrid approaches
Remuneration	Academic salary set by universities	NHS, private provider/organisation or local authority salary
Annual leave	Typically, 32 days with discretionary days	Varies
Pension	Teachers Pension Scheme or University Superannuation Scheme	NHS pension, Local Government Pension Scheme or pension dependent on private provider/organisation

Managing your diary as an educator/academic

The writers of this chapter are experienced academics who have been employed in a number of English universities and agree that diary management through a robust approach is essential; not only in meeting the needs of students and apprentices, but ensuring that there is a work-life balance.

Developing a healthy psychological contrast is a useful start in creating a strategy to managing your education/academic work, rather than being controlled by it. This can be achieved by replacing the word 'workload' with the word 'workstream', which may help in establishing a focus on productivity rather than mere labour. Here is one approach based on the use of an electronic diary, such as Microsoft Outlook:

Managing distinct workstreams

Use your electronic calendar to manage your work as well as appointments and meetings by scheduling work as either:

1 A **task** (taking less than half an hour).
2 An **activity** (taking an hour).
3 A **parcel of work** (taking more than an hour, a day or a number of days).

- Planned work can be moved, but only in accordance with the '**rule of three'**: a task, activity or parcel of work can be moved only up to three times before it must be completed. After all, procrastination is the thief of time … !
- Once a task, activity or parcel of work is completed, it should be marked [in the calendar] as 'DONE'. This is useful as it provides you with a sense of progression and achievement, particularly at the end of the day.
- Important work such as link lecturer/tutor visits or deadlines for marking may appear in the calendar in red-shaded boxes.

At the start of each week and during the week, the calendar should be reviewed with tasks, activities or parcels of work 'moved around' the calendar based on maximising your productivity. It is particularly useful if the allocation of work is made on the basis of high-intensity/demanding work at the start of the week, start of the day; and less demanding and intense work towards the end of the day or week. A useful analogy is that of an investment banker moving money around in order to get the best return on their investment.

- Large parcels of work, such as administration, lesson preparation, marking, educa-tional auditing, projects, research, scholarship and publication, should be planned months in advance.
- Important deadlines should be added in the diary using countdown notices, e.g. *'four weeks until article submission'; 'three weeks until NMC return'; 'A&E audit expires in two weeks'.*

Lastly, if you are permitted to work flexibly or in a hybrid manner, work-from-home days should be scheduled as a large parcel of work and should appear in the calendar as 'WFH' within the location box. This is particularly important as many employers expect their education/academic staff to demonstrate accountability for the use of their time, with line managers and heads of department requiring staff to 'share' their academic electronic calendar. Additionally, this may be a requirement of the employing organisa-tion's 'lone worker' policy, ensuring that the whereabouts of lone workers are known.

Strategy for appointments and management of meetings

All appointments and meetings can be scheduled using the electronic calendar with the 'meeting appointment request' e-mail function:

1 A **summary** or title of the meeting is provided.
2 The **name of person(s)** is included in the meeting invite or persons/colleagues accompanying.

3   The **location** of the meeting is included (room, building) and the post code (for those traveling by car and using satellite navigation systems).

Estimated travel time, typically in units of 30–60 minutes, can be entered within the calendar as 'travelling'. Recipients of meetings should be actively discouraged from emailing apologies in preference to either 'accepting' or 'declining' meetings in response to calendar invitations.

As an educator/academic, it is important to remember that your time belongs to you; it is yours to give away; if time is managed carefully, your time can be given away freely. Therefore, when arranging meetings off-site or -campus, an email with 'my availability' should be sent with perhaps no less than six suggested dates with particular times or simply 'AM/PM'. The scheduling of meetings on-site or -campus can be undertaken using a matrix for recipients to indicate their availability or even a 'Doodle Poll' [https://doodle.com/make-a-poll]

Managing emails

You may have noticed that we started this section by presenting a model of time management prior to the consideration of how best to manage emails. This is a reminder that education and academic practice requires more of a prospective, forward-facing strategic approach in comparison to clinical or practice settings, where a practitioner may be constantly reacting to patients' and clients' needs. Here is a suggested strategy for the management of emails:

- Only open an email twice; once to read it and respond immediately (if necessary); if not or the email is non-urgent, put it in the calendar as a task, activity or parcel of work.
- **'Let the world turn'** – most emails can wait, but be sure to acknowledge an email. It is good to indicate when you intend to 'action' the matter or when a parcel of work has been scheduled (in your calendar) for completion. This conveys to the recipient that you have recognised their needs and recognised the importance of the matter by making a time commitment with a cut-off date, e.g. '*I have ring-fenced time in my diary on … and hope to get back to you by the end of …*'
- Plan in your calendar time to deal with emails or time spent managing emails; again, as a task, activity or if you have just returned from leave, a parcel of work.

It is quite useful to schedule an email 'golden hour' at the start of each day or to schedule two 30-minute periods to keep on top of your emails. Lastly, whilst it is best practice to stay away from your emails when on holiday or on leave, some judicious 'housekeeping' of your email account by simply deleting spam or information-only emails can help when returning to work to what would otherwise be an unnecessarily large pile of emails.

Conclusion

This final chapter returned to the role of the practice supervisor, assessor and educator, but focused on the scope of practice whilst acknowledging the challenges of practice educators who fulfil a dual role. Our consideration of the core of steel needed to undertake assessment and the readiness of educators to do so was quite challenging as we saw that assessment practice is strongly related to values, beliefs and moral virtuosity as well as personality traits that may impinge on assessor readiness. Our case studies demonstrated the skills needed to supervise within advanced practice settings, as we saw with Sanjay, prior to a consideration of the role educational leadership. Tanya and Tom's case studies demonstrated the application of leadership in not only developing new practice education experiencing but delivering improvements to the practice setting that changed patient outcomes. Finally, our attention switched to opportunities for experienced supervisors, assessors and educators to transition to learning, teaching and academic roles and featured a comprehensive analysis of differences in working environments and strategies to successfully transition to the education/academic setting through the management of time, workstreams, meetings and emails.

A final word ...

We do hope that you have found *Practice Supervision and Assessment in Nursing, Health and Social Care* a useful and profitable read and that engagement with the activities enabled you to link the text to your own transformational learning experiences.

Our intention has been to identify the key themes, models and theoretical perspectives common to the supervision of students and apprentices within diverse practice learning settings and promote a trans-professional conversation of practice learning with reference to compassionate learning environments to promote the learning of all.

Our use of narratives, case studies and vignettes reminded the writing team of their indebtedness to successive mentors, educators, facilitators and lecturers, too numerous to mention, but the focus of our fond remembrance and for whom the book is dedicated.

Helpful resources

Chartered Society of Physiotherapy: https://www.csp.org.uk/publications/ahp-principles-practice-based-learning
Midlands, Yorkshire & East Practice Learning Group: https://myeweb.ac.uk/
Pan London Practice Learning Group: https://plplg.uk/
Pan London Practice Learning Group (Midwifery MORA): https://plplg.uk/emora/

References

Baluyot, CMA, Blomberg, K (2019) 'Challenges in assessment situations in clinical studies: How do nurse mentors in home-based health care services experience assessment situations in supervision of 2nd year bachelor nursing students?' *Nursing Primary Care*, 3 (1), pp. 1–8.
Barr, J, Dowding, L (2012) *Leadership in health care* (2nd ed.). London: Sage.
Brown, P, Jones, A, Davies, J (2020) 'Shall I tell my mentor? Exploring the mentor-student relationship and its impact on students' raising concerns on clinical placement', *Journal of Clinical Nursing*, 29, pp. 3298–3310. 10.1111/jocn.15356
CIPD (2023) *Leadership in the workplace: fact sheet*. London: Chartered Institute of Personnel & Development. Available at: https://www.cipd.org/uk/knowledge/factsheets/leadership-factsheet/
CODP (2021) *Standards for supporting pre-registration operating department practitioner education in practice placements*. Available at: https://www.unison.org.uk/content/uploads/2021/12/CODP-Standards-for-Supporting-Pre-Registration-Operating-Department-Practitioner-Education-in-Practice-Placements-December-2021.pdf

Gallagher, A (2006) 'Promoting ethical competence', in David, AJ, Tschudin, V, De Raeve, L (eds), *The teaching of nursing ethics: Content and methods*. Edinburgh: Elsevier, pp. 223–239.

HEE (2017) *Multi-professional framework for advanced clinical practice in England*. London: Health Education England. Available at: https://www.hee.nhs.uk/sites/default/files/documents/multi-professionalframeworkforadvancedclinicalpracticeinengland.pdf

Helminen, K, Coco, K, Johnson, M, Turimen, Tossavainen, K (2016) 'Summative assessment of clinical practice of student nurses: A review of the literature', *International Journal of Nursing Studies*, 53, pp. 308–319.

Hunt, LA (2019) 'Developing a "core of steel": The key attributes of effective practice assessors', *British Journal of Nursing*, 28 (22), pp. 1478–1484.

Mullins, L (2004) *Management & organisational behaviour* (7th ed.). Harlow: Prentice Hall.

NMC (2023) *Standards for student supervision and assessment*. Available at: https://www.nmc.org.uk/standards-for-education-and-training/standards-for-student-supervision-and-assessment/

Index